A
NEW
PERCEPTION

Dedicated to the children and parents
who allowed me into their lives

A NEW PERCEPTION

OF THE EVOLUTION
OF HUMAN BEHAVIOUR
AND ITS DISORDERS

ROBERT BUGLER
F.R.C.PSYCH., M.R.C.G.P.

ISBN (Paperback): 978-1-912892-40-2
ISBN (eBook): 978-1-912892-41-9

Project management by whitefox
Designed and typeset by seagulls.net
Cover design by Madeline Meckiffe

CONTENTS

ABOUT THIS BOOK

Compared to the dramatic advances made in every other branch of medicine, psychiatry has been unable to make significant progress for half a century. Psychiatry, or the study of disordered behaviour, is ultimately a subdivision of behavioural science that has never identified basic phenomena akin to the laws of physics and elements in chemistry that brought success in those fields. In short, psychiatry has not moved forward because the simplest forms of behaviour or 'responses to change in the environment' have not been identified and the law-like precepts that have shaped their evolution have not been recognized. The knowledge is 'out there' but has never been brought together in a coherent system.

A New Perception unravels a small group of elemental behaviours that arise from and reinforce unicellular physiology. They continue throughout animal life and recent evidence shows that they contribute to our mental and physical health. Unfortunately, the functional adaptations that have contributed to human intelligence and ability have brought instabilities that we experience as mental illnesses.

INTRODUCTION

This work was initially prompted by my failure to protect a child from further harm during court proceedings in 1977. The High Court judge dismissed my evidence by asserting that psychiatry had no scientific basis. I was frustrated because I had failed and because he was right.

I tried to persuade fellow psychiatrists that, compared to the dramatic advances in other medical fields, the specialty was hardly making any progress. It was very foolish of me; if my comment registered at all it made me unpopular, but it usually fell on deaf ears.

* * *

During the past forty years, neurology, the study and treatment of physical disorders in the brain, spinal cord and nerves, has made extraordinary progress, facilitated by the invention and use of very sophisticated instruments. Our knowledge of cerebral function, of the biochemical changes that take place in the brain and of the transmission of impulses has increased immensely. Unfortunately, the complex research has not brought any meaningful advance in the prevention and treatment of mental illness.

In summary, mental illnesses remain largely unexplained and the way in which medication and other therapies alleviate the different conditions has not been resolved.

In reading Thomas Kuhn's *The Structure of Scientific Revolutions*, and encouraged by a phone call from the author, I became convinced that the only way in which progress might be gained was to start with the most elemental behavioural phenomena that could be identified. It has taken many years to discriminate the simplest 'responses to change'. I have been surprised to find that fulfilling those behaviours contributes to our mental and physical health.

I have been left in no doubt by my former colleagues that they consider the concept a fantasy. They are unable to comprehend the reconception because some behavioural phenomena are given different interpretations to their established beliefs.

A radical revision is never easy to assimilate; the work is set out in as user-friendly language as possible and directed first to lay readers, with references to easily accessible sources like Wikipedia, in the hope that they will urge the profession to move on from their present beliefs and assumptions.

PERSONAL NOTE

Like many children who grew up during the disruptive experiences of the Second World War, I had little self-confidence so I could hardly believe it when I was accepted as a student at St Bartholomew's Hospital Medical School.

Possibly through the gratitude that I felt, I took the words of Sir James Paterson Ross, spoken on my first day at medical school, to heart. The new students were assembled in the Great Hall of the hospital, which was lined with portraits of Henry VIII, the patron of the hospital and its distinguished physicians and surgeons. Sir Paterson Ross, then surgeon to King George VI, gave a short speech. He welcomed us and said that we were privileged to study at and be part of the hospital where William Harvey had first resolved the cardiovascular circulation. He urged us not to let our predecessors down, and to act at all times in the interests of our patients.

This is a final attempt to fulfil that responsibility.

* * *

My years as a medical student were followed by appointment as a house physician at St Bartholomew's. It was the busiest but most fulfilling year of my life.

After three years of National Service in a peacetime Royal Navy, I became an assistant in general practice, but found my obstetric experience inadequate and undertook a short obstetric appointment. From 1961 to 1970 I was a single-handed general practitioner.

Through unusual circumstances I transferred (with some disapproval of psychiatric colleagues) directly to a consultant child and adolescent psychiatrist appointment. I ended my career privileged and inspired to be working at Sheffield Children's University Teaching Hospital.

CHAPTER 1

'ANOTHER ATTEMPT'

This concept has evolved over thirty years; I have made many attempts to arouse interest and expose it to criticism without success, and became resigned to failure. But on 28 December 2017 the BBC broadcast two television programmes.

On BBC Two, David Attenborough recorded the behaviour of wood ants who live in unusually large and successful colonies. In those colonies, individuals with different genetic identities live together without seeking to eradicate each other. He noted that the behaviour was unusual and (biological) rethinking might be necessary.

A little earlier, on BBC Four, in a Christmas lecture from the Royal Society, Professor Sophie Scott demonstrated that many animals communicate through body language and sounds but cannot combine multiple pieces of information into the single communication that humans have achieved: e.g. 'A mile after passing the left turn to Dingley village, turn right up an unmarked lane.'

The larger size of human brains did not, in her opinion, sufficiently explain greater human ability but it was possible that we had a different – human – 'operating system'.

This minute shift by two established authorities on critical evolutionary points and some filling in of gaps since my last attempt have persuaded me to try to achieve publication once more.

* * *

Even within the profession, the absence of progress has been noted for decades but not addressed.

In 2003 the retiring editor of the *British Journal of Psychiatry* was asked, 'Do you think that psychiatry and psychiatric research are any further forward?' He replied, 'Not much, if at all; and, in clinical settings, there has been a deterioration.' More recently, in January 2018, the current editor wrote: 'Outcomes in psychosis are disheartening. We know this as clinicians and we have all had patients for whom our best efforts appear to be failing' and later in the same editorial 'that stumped feeling when people ask "Yeah but how does it [electroconvulsive therapy, ECT] work?"'[1]

On 11 November 2018, the *Spectator* reprinted the winning John Murray prize essay by Taj Nathan, an eminent forensic psychiatrist. In the exceptional essay he states, 'the more I have examined the criminal manifestations of the human mind, the more I have seen the limitations of medical diagnosis', and he concludes that 'the physiology of the brain has to be contextualized by psychological abstractions of the mind such as impulses, urges, motives and inhibitions'. In other words, human behaviour will never be successfully elucidated solely through biochemical and electronic measurement.

Possibly those most disenchanted with psychiatry are consultants in other medical specialties; surgeons in particular will denigrate psychiatry in private. One reason for their disregard is that the specialty has no coherent system.

Psychiatrists, and others who care for the mentally ill, work as hard and are as committed to their patients as surgeons and physicians – but they are not serving their patients' interests by failing to confront the lack of progress.

* * *

During ten years as a family doctor I saw forty or more families at home every week. There was a wide variety of child caring, most

---

[1] Also 'The treatment of schizophrenia has hardly changed in the past fifty years and depression scarcely in the past twenty', Nesse, R. M., *Good Reasons for Bad Feelings: Insights from the Frontier of Evolutionary Psychiatry* (London: Allen Lane, 2019). Quoted in *The British Journal of General Practice*, 2019, 69: pp 105–106.

loving, a few abusive. I entered my new profession without special-
ized training, without having acquired attachment to one or other
of the schools of thought. I followed the methods that my colleagues
advanced with less than total conviction. I found the most successful management of any case depended upon a careful history of the
events that had preceded a child's change of behaviour.

Medication was rarely of any help. The most successful outcome
happened when parents felt that they had, themselves, restored
family well-being.

ADAM[2]

Once they knew what was necessary, many parents understood better
than I did what should be done. Adam's mother brought him to see
me because his character had changed after falling down a bank and
suffering several injuries. He had become very anxious, complained
of symptoms that had no physical signs and was reluctant to go out.
When I asked what had happened before he had fallen, his mother
replied, 'That's an interesting question. A day or two before he fell
he was a server at communion in church for the first time. He made
many mistakes and was roundly told off by our elderly priest.'

After gaining Adam's confidence, he told me that he had made
so many mistakes in church, he was certain God had punished him
by pushing him down the bank. God was only waiting for a similar
opportunity to finish him off.

The solution was much easier than in many other cases. Adam's
mother settled on the remedy herself. She arranged for a young priest
to have Adam as a server to give him practice, praise and reassurance.

* * *

By 1983, I was frustrated by the absence of any coherent system
of behaviour that I believed must exist and concluded that such

---

[2] With one exception, all names have been changed.

a system could only be unravelled by starting with the simplest of behavioural phenomena. I had no idea how far back that would take me.

I happened to read an article in the *Economist* that brought Professor Kuhn's *The Structure of Scientific Revolutions* to my notice and I borrowed the essay from the university library.

Whilst working at MIT in 1961, Thomas Kuhn reviewed the past history of scientific discoveries to prepare lecture notes for non-scientific students. He was astonished by the consistent circumstances that had occurred whenever a significant advance had been achieved. The revolutionary event was preceded by competing schools of thought and a period without progress. Success came from discarding established convictions, by reconceiving the field from its most basic phenomena and by introducing material from other disconnected fields. He noted that the established authorities in a field had never been able to carry out the necessary reconception – or relate to it when it had occurred.

This work attempts to reproduce a Kuhnian reconception, which he labelled a 'paradigm'.[3]

* * *

Psychiatry is ultimately a subdivision of behavioural science. Behavioural science records the reactions of species and gives labels to the events. Further interest in any phenomenon is restricted to the contribution the particular behaviour makes to survival, procreation and social existence.

Any successful reconception of psychiatry has to separate from the established interpretations of behaviour by behavioural scientists.

---

[3] 'The paradigm functions by permitting the replication of examples any one of which could in principle serve to replace it.' And later on the same page, 'We must recognize how very limited in both scope and precision a paradigm can be at the time of its first appearance. Paradigms gain their status because they are more successful than their competitors in solving a few problems that the group of practitioners has come to recognize as acute.' Kuhn, Thomas S., *The Structure of Scientific Revolutions* (University of Chicago Press, Third Edition, 1996) p 23.

Reconception is unavoidably an anathema to academics and those immersed in the current constructs of behaviour and mental illness. However, if the iron grip of Darwinian evolution on the generation and development of behaviour is slightly relaxed, the system that surfaces provides solutions to some unanswered questions. A rational origin of the autonomic nervous system unfolds and fragile developmental periods that make autism and ADHD (Attention Deficit Hyperactivity Disorder) possible are exposed. The final evolutionary step explains our human susceptibility to unhappiness, self-harm and suicide.

CHAPTER 2

BARRIERS TO RECONCEPTION

Four major factors hinder moving on from current behavioural concepts.

1. The dominance of natural selection.
2. The constant flood of new information.
3. The artificial invention – verbal language – which is unreliable in defining emotions, motivations and dysfunctions.
4. Absence of alternative.

1. NATURAL SELECTION

The concept of survival, through competition between individuals and species, is rational and demonstrable in every natural environment.

This work does not deny the influence of evolution on motivation to survive or that it dominates animal and, occasionally, human lives. When fire, flood or other disasters threaten we can all be driven to ignore others and attempt to escape, but these are rare events that many never experience. It is irrational to accept that human lives are subject to and function with a system focused upon events that seldom happen.

The autocracy of natural selection is evident in many natural history programmes broadcast on television. Strange forms of behaviour are recorded and the viewer's interest is aroused. Every debate that follows such a presentation is solely confined to which aspect of survival will profit most from the phenomenon. It is never posited that the behaviour could be interpreted in a different context. The biological school of behaviour resembles a juggernaut that blocks any other concept but completely fails to elucidate most human behaviour.

* * *

Behaviour, however, arose before competition, before the semi-conscious drive to survive emerged.

It arose from cellular physiology and was directed towards protecting biochemical reactions and the other functions that maintain life. The primitive forms of response, of behaviour and the evolutionary precepts became established and continued throughout animal and our own evolution.

When multicellular life arose and flourished, physiology was more efficiently maintained by allocating separate metabolic responsibilities to groups of cells in different organs. The vital processes ceased to be vulnerable and the first **purpose** of behaviour, the protection of cellular physiology, became redundant. It created a void that was replaced by competitive survival.

After a billion years, through the acquisition of intelligence and greater adaptability, competitive survival ceased to be as stimulating a challenge for our hominid ancestors, threatening another void. A more compelling alternative evolved – and dominates our lives.

2. THE CONSTANT FLOOD OF INFORMATION

If I suggested that psychiatry was not making much progress to a colleague, they would point to more than forty English-language psychiatric journals and the desperate struggle by many to have their research published.

This confuses activity with progress. In the absence of a coherent system, the mass of academic papers makes it almost impossible to separate significant work from the more routine.

3. VERBAL LANGUAGE

The language that we use is artificial. It has shaped our lives and behaviour ever since it was extended from simple sounds.

Its inadequacy is recognized but not acted upon. Albert Ellis and Robert Harper[1] summarize the situation:

> 'Man is a uniquely language-creating animal and he
> begins to learn from very early childhood to formulate
> his thoughts, perceptions and feelings in words, phrases
> and sentences. If this is so and we have no evidence to
> the contrary, then for all practical purposes the phrases
> and sentences that we keep telling ourselves usually are or
> become our thoughts and emotions.'

Others note that differing language and culture change the character of human behaviour. Jenny Yiend, Bundy Mackintosh and George Savulch in 'Cognition and Emotion'[2] state:

> 'To complicate matters, different languages and cultures
> do seem to differ in the number and categorization of their
> emotion terms. It is not surprising to find that the range
> of situations that trigger emotions varies across cultures
> but in addition, different emotions are either elaborated or
> downgraded in emphasis. These data support the idea that
> emotional vocalizations are recognized across cultures but
> that differences in language have an effect.'

It is inescapable that human behaviour is modified by our artificial language. We could be said to live a theatrical script that directs our

---

[1] Ellis, Albert and Harper, Robert, 'A Guide to Rational Living', in Butler-Bowdon, Tom, ed., *50 Psychology Classics* (Nicholas Brealey Publishing, 2012) p 74.
[2] In Braisby, Nick and Gellatly, Angus, eds., *Cognitive Psychology* (OUP, 2nd Edition, 2012) p 518.

behaviour and responses; behaviour that may not coincide with any inherent 'operating system'.

The present situation makes it essential to move away from behaviour derived from the communal script, to identify basic phenomena and ensure that any labels given to those phenomena are as simple as possible.

In this work, we have very few attributes and very few emotional responses but language separates both into many different entities. For example, mischief is considered later in this work to be an attribute of acting out of character to unsettle other people; it ranges from practical jokes to serial killing. If I try to convey that single interpretation to others, I am told that the first is a poor sense of humour and the latter is just evil. We should not reject the possibility that perpetrators enjoy the same satisfaction in causing dismay, because their actions and satisfactions are so widely different in degree.

4. ABSENCE OF ALTERNATIVE

No one seeks an alternative until it is recognized that a field is faltering. Even if doubts arise, current convictions must persist until an alternative concept is available. *A New Perception* provides one; there may be others.

CHAPTER 3

CONFLICTING SCHOOLS

There are three 'schools' that influence psychiatry. Each one has value and useful therapeutic strategies. If candidates for a consultant post are asked which school they follow, they can reply that they are eclectic and use whichever method is most likely to be successful for any particular patient.

In minimal categorization, the three schools are:

1. 'Behaviourist', which follows the work of Pavlov, who trained dogs to look for and expect food when he rang a bell. In other words, we learn to associate events: an infant, for example, anticipates going out when she/he is put into warm clothes.

   In a television programme, Professor Ian Robertson demonstrated subtle behaviourist therapy when he coaxed a journalist fearful of travelling down a zip wire to rethink the event. She was urged to avoid focusing on the height above ground and any apparent danger but to look upon the event and imitate the body language of one taking part in a new and exciting experience. It was very successful; she was delighted to have had the thrill that she had feared. The striking experiment demonstrated that self-limiting anxieties and behaviour can be displaced by changing the subject's perception of events.

2. 'Psychoanalysis'. Sigmund Freud established that we have subconscious mental activity that can affect our emotional

stability through internal conflicts, unsatisfied desires or the repression of memory of untoward experiences. The subconscious can influence our responses and our attitude to others. His method of therapy can be life-changing but like any powerful therapy it can harm if therapists are insufficiently trained.

3. The third and dominant school is the Darwinian: 'Biological'. It is well known that physical or somatic changes arise through genetic variation. If the changes are advantageous, they are perpetuated by natural selection. Those who subscribe to the biological school believe that the same path has shaped human as well as animal behaviour.

* * *

Any system must have both a purpose or goal and precepts (rules of action) through which it evolves and functions. The cardiovascular system, for example, is a transport system. Its purpose is to carry fluid and nutrients throughout the body and carry metabolites (waste products) away. To function efficiently, like any pump and circulatory system, the precepts are: (a) fluid must not leak before entering capillaries; (b) pressure must not fluctuate excessively; (c) the lining of the vessels has to be smooth; and (d) blood viscosity is reasonably constant.

To recapitulate, the essential first step in making any system intelligible must be to identify the rules or precepts that give it order.

CHAPTER 4

THE ORIGINAL PURPOSE AND PRECEPTS OF THE BEHAVIOURAL SYSTEM

Behaviour, or the response to change in the environment, could not have arisen 'out of the blue'. Logically, the only resource behaviour could have evolved from was internal cellular activity or cellular physiology and the only initial purpose of the response could be protection and reinforcement of that physiology.

There is need in every scientific system to discover the most elemental or irreducible particles or phenomena. In unravelling behaviour, elemental phenomena can be discerned in bacteria and unicellular life forms.

Many will consider it insane to propose that human behaviour is in any way related to bacterial behaviour but it has already been noted that many of the metabolic processes that keep us alive were established in nucleated bacteria.

Cellular behaviour evolved from cellular physiology, which functions within three 'precepts':

1. A stable internal state (homeostasis) is essential to living cells.
2. A changing external environment is equally vital.

And almost as dominant as the first two:

3. Nature is unfailingly economic, which has consequences:

a) Every new advance is built upon resources already established.

b) Every function has to be exercised occasionally for it to remain available. Nature does not allow passengers; if an organ or function is not utilized it gradually degenerates and can be lost.

1. MAINTAINING A STEADY INTERNAL STATE WITHIN THE CELL

The 'father of physiology', Claude Bernard (1813–1878), first recognized the necessity for cells to maintain their internal condition in a balanced steady state; in other words, the constituents of a cell and its biochemical activity are limited to minimal variation. His words were: '*La fixité du milieu intérieur est la condition de la vie libre.*' ('Internal stability is essential to the living condition.')[1]

Walter Cannon (1871–1945), of the Harvard Medical School, labelled the activity 'homeostasis' in 1932.[2]

The function of every cell in our bodies is to maintain a balanced, intracellular state.

2. CONSTANT CONDITIONS LEAD TO ABNORMAL DEVELOPMENT, DISEASE AND EVEN DEATH[3]

Every cell needs a changing external environment to exercise, to maintain the activity that ensures homeostasis.

The environment, the climate, temperature, barometric pressure, moisture fluctuates for most animals, including ourselves, without effort. That is less certain for micro-organisms: instead, bacteria have evolved flagella and ciliates have a fur-like covering

---

[1]   https://en.wikipedia.org/wiki/Milieu_intérieur
[2]   https://en.wikipedia.org/wiki/Walter_Bradford_Cannon
[3]   Koukkari, Willard L. and Sothern, Robert B., *Introducing Biological Rhythms* (Springer Science, 2006) p 48.

that enable them to achieve change through movement. Halobacteria have gas vacuoles, which convey them from the bottom to the surface of stagnant, high-salinity pools.

3. A) ORGANS AND FUNCTIONS ARE ECONOMICALLY DEVELOPED FROM RESOURCES THAT HAVE ALREADY BEEN ESTABLISHED

The process is colourfully described by Professor Brian Cox: 'Evolution is sometimes less of a watchmaker than a tinkering odd job man with oily overalls and a dirty face, mixing as best he can to get a job done by modifying the available parts.'[4]

A striking example occurs in the evolution from fish to reptiles and mammals. The gill arches become modified to pharyngeal, mandibular and inner ear structures, changing structure and function. That redeployment (ontogeny) of structure and function is fleetingly played out in the development of the human embryo.

B) EVERY ORGAN AND FUNCTION MUST BE EXERCISED TO CONTINUE TO EXIST: 'AS WITH ANY BIOLOGICAL FUNCTION, A LACK OF USE LEADS TO ATROPHY'[5]

One example, amongst many, of degeneration associated with lack of use is that the optic lobe of the brain in small blind crustaceans that live without light is much reduced.[6]

A more interesting example from our own lives is loss of the first language acquired by a child that happens after living in and only using the language of a second country. It is called 'language attrition'.

---

[4] Cox, Brian and Cohen, Andrew, *Wonders of Life* (Collins, 2013) p 183.
[5] Lipton, Bruce H., *The Biology of Belief* (Hay House; 10th Anniversary edition, 2015).
[6] http://www.biomedcentral.com/1471-2202/16/19

CHAPTER 5

ELEMENTAL BEHAVIOURS

Many attempts are made to define the emotions that we experience; for example, love and disgust. Dictionaries struggle to convey the feelings. From Chambers Dictionary:

Love: fondness, charity, an affection for something that gives pleasure, devoted attachment to another person.

Disgust: a loathing, distaste, extreme disapproval or annoyance.

The difficulty arises because the complex emotions are not single entities but combinations of elemental perceptions and responses. The first rational step in unravelling behavioural phenomena must be to identify seven irreducible responses, responses that cannot be further simplified that occur in the most primitive organisms.

1. CELLULAR OSCILLATION

Bacteria, unicellular life and all nucleated living cells oscillate and the oscillation is 'energized' when there is change in the cell's environment.

Cellular oscillation was established by Brian Goodwin (1931–2009) in 1965, whilst working at MIT.[1] In his paper, Professor

---

[1] Goodwin, Brian, 'A Statistical Mechanics of Temporal Organization in Cells', presented at the Society for Experimental Biology Symposium and published in its Journal, No 18, 1965, pp 301–326.

Goodwin demonstrated that all cells in animal organisms oscillate and the activity facilitates homeostasis, vital to cellular physiology.

If oscillation is interrupted, cells cannot survive. Professor Goodwin also recorded that the oscillation adjusts to stimuli: in an equable environment, it is a fine vibration. When the environment alters, both rhythm of oscillation and biochemical balance are inducted more powerfully to avoid internal function being disrupted – alternatively, any fluctuation of oscillation in the cell affects the biochemical, homeostatic balance and vice versa.

As there is little general awareness of homeostasis, and even less of cellular oscillation, an analogy could help. Consider a tennis match in which the core activity is keeping the ball in the air (homeostasis) and not allowing it to fade to the ground or fly from the court. When either the motion of the ball in the air or the return rhythm changes, it provokes a more active and purposeful oscillation between the players. When return is in accord there is less stimulus and less need for it to be dynamic.[2]

Human emotions parallel the cellular oscillatory reaction to change, to events. We are 'aroused' by social or material change in our environment. The greater the degree of change or significance of an event, the greater the arousal.

---

[2] The presence of oscillation in bacteria and the cells of living tissues is established but the following may more clearly reveal the close association between oscillation and physiological processes. From *Scientific American* 'Ask the Experts' April 3 2006: 'Why do cats purr?' Cats purr during both inhalation and exhalation with a consistent pattern and frequency between 25 and 150 Hertz. Various investigators have shown that the sound frequencies in this range improve bone density and promote healing. See also 'High frequency oscillation in patients with acute lung injury (ARDS) reduces hospital or 30-day mortality and improves oxygenation', BMJ2010;340:c2327 doi: 10.1136/bmj.c2327.

2. BIOLOGICAL RHYTHMS

We have at least 214 biological rhythms operating within us; we are aware of menstruation, cardiac, respiratory and sleep rhythms,[3] but completely unaware of many others. They often influence our perception and response.

Biological rhythms could not have evolved without underlying cellular oscillation. (Precept 3, page 18.)

Biological rhythms enable the essential processes to rotate, making more economic use of the limited space and resources of a single cell. They can be compared to a factory shift system, servicing machinery at night when there is no need to undertake work relating to the external environment: c.f. materials entering, goods leaving.[4]

It follows that disruption – the disorganization of biological rhythms – could be damaging but human biological rhythms have remarkable characteristics:

a) They can control us: if the rhythm or need to sleep becomes dominant it will overwhelm us no matter how hard we try to keep awake.

b) We can interrupt rhythms for short and occasionally long periods. For example, hold our breath, force ourselves to stay awake.

c) External events can interrupt rhythms: personal tragedies make sleep impossible.

---

[3] Humans and other animals have genetically based biological clocks that are present in individual cells, resulting in semi-autonomous oscillators in many peripheral tissues that can be coordinated by the suprachiasmic nucleus in the anterior hypothalamus. See Koukkari, Willard L. and Sothern, Robert B., *Introducing Biological Rhythms* (Springer Science, 2006) p 433.

[4] Zada, D., Bronshtein, I., Lerer-Goldshtein, T., Garini Y. and Appelbaum, L., 'Sleep increases chromosome dynamics to enable reduction of accumulating DNA damage in single neurons', *Nature Communications*, Volume 10, Article number: 895 (2019). DOI https://doi.org/10.1038/s41467-019-08806-w

And notoriously in human lives, a particular adaptability we make use of:

d) We can modify or entrain rhythms to coincide with external events. Those who travel widely adjust sleep to coincide with local time.

Some biological rhythms directly influence our behaviour. Two that are often evident to family members or co-workers are changes of mood associated with:

i)   Insulin secretion, which is highest in the afternoon and reduces blood glycogen. We can be less alert and less amenable when glycogen is low.
ii) Premenstrual[5] involuntary mood changes.

Our diurnal rhythms also affect our resilience: onset of toothache is most common in the early morning, osteoarthritic pain in the knee is greatest in the evening and the most intense episodes of angina occur between 2 a.m. and 6 a.m.[6]

There is damage – a physiological price to pay – if endogenous cycles are persistently dislocated, repeatedly forced to adapt. When rhythms of sleep and wakefulness are constantly disrupted, physical and cognitive functions deteriorate, leading to ill health.[7]

Biological rhythms orchestrate and maintain physiological processes; they influence our behaviour. We use their adaptability and manipulate them to satisfy artificially contrived circumstances, night-time employment and air travel.

[5] Louann Brizendine was struck by the extent to which the female brain is shaped by dramatic changes in hormonal chemistry, driving a woman's behaviour and creating her reality. See Brizendine, Louann, 'The Female Brain', in Butler-Bowdon, Tom, ed., *50 Psychology Classics* (Nicholas Brealey Publishing, 2012) p 53.
[6] Koukkari, Willard L. and Sothern, Robert B., *Introducing Biological Rhythms* (Springer Science, 2006) p 443.
[7] Disruption of the normal circadian clock may promote carcinogenesis. Ibid. p 487.

3. EMOTIONAL RESPONSE

Both extreme environmental change and no change are inimical to microscopic life. In addition, some slight changes can affect vital processes; a trace amount of copper is, for example, lethal to marine invertebrates.

The possibility of small amounts of toxic substances entering the environment created a need for the sensory attributes that preceded smell, taste, touch and hearing in our lives. There is evidence of early sensory ability in unicellular forms when they move to the most hospitable accessible sites, but microscopic life responds first to the volume or quantity of environmental change:

a) Too small to stimulate oscillation; i.e., no response.
b) A volume that stimulates oscillation favourably.
c) A large enough volume to require oscillatory compensation.
d) A damaging volume or extent of change – lethal unless it can be separated from.

In our lives we are also initially aroused by the 'volume' of environmental and social change but unless it is or appears to be d) a disaster, arousal is followed in milliseconds by distinguishing its congenial or uncongenial nature and we respond accordingly. In short, for all practical purposes response is fashioned by emotional decisions[8] – by how we characterize any event, as with the journalist and the zip wire above (page 14).

In academic literature, research into emotions has been hampered by focusing on the physical components of an event (sound, light, texture, movement) and a misleading search for a survival advantage as an explanation for the introduction of emotion. In reality, as

---

[8] The difference in volume of sound of a kettle about to boil over alerts us but we immediately focus on its advantage in bringing a cup of tea nearer, or disadvantage in that it will 'boil over'.

oscillation changes with every event, emotion and cognition occur at virtually the same time.[9]

We are not conscious of internal oscillatory change (though our pulse rate and blood pressure often increase) but we can be aware of the biochemical change that accompanies an arousing or stimulating event. It is referred to as an adrenaline rush and occurs whenever a particularly pleasant or unpleasant event is anticipated.

In this evolution of behaviour, response is founded in cellular physiology. Change in the external environment is either '**hospitable**' to a cell's physiology or '**inhospitable**'. Those convenient **generic** labels are carried forward in this evolution, eventually to our own lives where hospitable social events or contacts enhance our sense or our image of ourselves (which replaces physiology as the point about which human response pivots) and inhospitable occasions diminish it.

When a significant event has occurred a more powerful oscillation[10] is aroused and, as with a pendulum, it must continue until the energy is expended through redirection, friction or other abatement. If it is not expended, like an orchestral percussionist who fails to dampen his kettledrum, the residual sound waves intrude upon the following music. If we fail to move our thoughts on from a stimulating experience, the emotion or oscillation interferes with our ability to appreciate and respond equally to further events. Pragmatically, we dampen ongoing arousal by dissipating it through cheering, clapping, swearing, hugging and many other actions. Chimpanzees and children chatter, dogs wag their tails.

If a close friend dies, for example, we are compelled to tell other people in order to lose some of the arousal as soon as possible. It is more difficult to move on from some untoward events, such as

---

[9] Recent research has moved towards a construct that coincides with such a proposition, with emotional events being placed on an affect grid having a 'positive/ negative' categorization axis and a 'calm/aroused' (or volume of arousal) axis. Braisby, Nick and Gellatly, Angus, eds., *Cognitive Psychology* (OUP, Second Edition, 2012) p 519.

[10] In the brain and evident from electroencephalograms.

having a fall or losing a wallet. They cause a continuing oscillation or distraction that makes it more likely that we will have another accident or mislay another object.

Much of human life is directed towards enjoying change that engenders arousal. We seek variety in food, clothes, companions, etc. We pay large sums to experience holidays through tedious airports and in hotels less comfortable than our own homes just to have stimulating change.[11]

Change in the external environment is resolved through tactile and chemical senses[12] that have developed from cellular oscillation and homeostasis. It is characterized emotionally (hospitable or inhospitable) and is followed by a momentum related to significance of the event.

4. MOTILITY

When there is no change, when an environment is static, oscillation is not stimulated. The evolution of flagella and cilia in microscopic life enabled micro-organisms to move and through that to experience change. Recurrent or continuous motility became an essential activity for cells, including those of higher forms of life. It continues to be achieved by moving as an individual in the environment or inducing the environment to flow past. Reptiles, birds and mammals constantly move the external environment through in respiration and maintain internal flow by their vascular and lymphatic systems. In other words, motility, like the many extensions of oscillatory rhythms, is extended into several conscious and unconscious functions.

In our lives we move, physically or psychologically, towards whatever we find hospitable and away from the inhospitable. We

---

[11] 'Neophilia' underlies the foundation of art, music, television, film, publishing, drug taking, travel, pornography and fashion. Whiten, A. and Byrne, R. W., eds., *Machiavellian Intelligence II* (Cambridge University Press, 1997) p 331.

[12] Chemical changes that permeate from the external environment will affect cellular biochemistry whilst any physical change that intrudes will affect oscillation.

can simulate movement by travelling in vehicles and in our imag-
ination. The beneficial effects for health of actual movement, of
undertaking exercise, are recognized in an abundance of studies.[13] At
the other extreme, hours of sensory deprivation can end in mental
disorder. (From Wikipedia: '… extended or forced sensory deprivation can result in extreme anxiety, hallucinations, bizarre thoughts
and depression.'[14])

**The need to experience change (precept 2, page 17) is satis-
fied by movement through the environment or moving the
environment past, both in single cells and the cells of multicellular life forms.**

Recapitulation

I have attempted to show that human arousal parallels the characteristics of cellular oscillation. In addition, the more significant or
dramatic an event, the more powerful the continuing momentum
– or mental preoccupation with what has recently happened.

I have also attempted to show that biological rhythms are as
vital to us as they are to unicellular life and that disordering the
rhythms can damage our health.

Changing the environment and movement helps to maintain
health whilst our well-being deteriorates with insufficient exercise.

In summary, the 'elemental' behaviours that have been set out
reinforce both cellular physiology and human health.

5. ALTERNATE SELVES

There is a remarkable phenomenon or 'response to change' of unicellular life that evolves into an influential system of multicellular life.

---

[13] Amongst many other reports, the *Proceedings of the National Academy for Sciences
of the United States of America*, 2011, doi:10.1073/pnas.1015950108, showed
that older adults who walked for 40 minutes three times a week increased their
brain volume and memory, including improvements in spatial memory.
[14] https://en.wikipedia.org/wiki/Sensory_deprivation

The response is vital to bacterial survival and the system it engenders has been the subject of many studies. I have not found evidence that the two have previously been connected.

The elemental behaviour may be more easily understood by looking back from human habits to the response in unicellular life.

Mammalian hibernation, sleep and recurrent depression have a common characteristic: they all separate the individual from the environment – in depression, from the social environment. A sense of detachment is not a headline symptom of depression but those who are affected will often say they feel cut off from others. Individuals who live with a depressed relative frequently comment that he or she is difficult to communicate with.

Being separate or self-contained is involuntary in depression but we can all wish from time to time, like unicellular organisms, to be just ourselves. That we could 'have our own space' and be in charge of our lives, free of responsibility to anyone else, their influence or their intrusion – and we may arrange to satisfy that urge.[15]

In accord with precept 3 (page 18), involuntary self-containment in depression and the relatively common voluntary self-containment must have had a precursor. It can be found in bacterial and unicellular life.

When there is overwhelming change in the external environment, micro-organisms undergo a dramatic metamorphosis: they become 'spores'. In spore form, a micro-organism has an insulating coat that separates it from the external environment and makes it impervious to extreme cold and heat, strong acids and alkalis.

Textbooks such as one written by James Hoch in 1976 state that: sporulation also 'commences at the end of exponential growth

---

[15] Greta Garbo, film star of the 1930s: 'I never said, "I want to be alone." I only said, "I want to be left alone." There is all the difference.' She retired from the screen, at the age of 35, after acting in 28 films and from then on, Garbo declined all opportunities to return to the screen. Shunning publicity, she began a private life (Wikipedia, https://en.wikipedia.org/wiki/Greta_Garbo).

in a culture'.[16] I believe this should read instead: 'sporulation ends exponential growth in a culture because sporulation behaviour has to be exercised from time to time to ensure that the facility is not lost.' In effect there is, even in hospitable circumstances, a need to 'exercise' the 'separating' behaviour to prevent degradation.

Although it is a remarkable 'response to change', biologists do not identify the metamorphic process as a behavioural event but focus upon the ability of spores to survive and the fact that the phenomenon is a path to asexual reproduction.

Evolution to multicellular life with protective coatings – e.g. shells, exoskeletons, skin – superseded the need for sporulation but it is unthinkable that nature would squander such a valuable resource, and it has moved to rotation between two behavioural conditions:

i)   Open to the external environment, freely exchanging gases and metabolites with the external environment.

ii) Closed, separated from, having reduced interaction with the external environment.

Both conditions are fundamental behavioural states that figure extensively in this concept – generic conditions that do not currently have a specific name. It will be easier and less cluttering to the text to give them labels:

i)   **Apertic**, from the Latin *apertus* – 'open door' = open, expansive and active upon the external environment, engaged in pursuing evolutionary purpose.

ii) **Recedic**, from the Latin *recedum* – 'shrinking from duty' = closed in upon oneself, separated from the external environment as far as

---

[16] Hoch, James A., 'Genetics of Bacterial Sporulation', *Advances in Genetics*, Vol 18, 1976, pp 69–98. It is interesting to note that temporal sequences of morphological and biochemical events are quite similar to the ordered sequences that characterize the development of higher organisms. Similar physiologies might be expected to have similar responses to change.

possible, a response brought about by the inhospitableness of the external environment. The evolutionary purpose is relinquished.

An evolutionary change that transformed a metamorphic event into an adaptable behaviour would need spores to be incorporated, at some time, into the cell tissues and there is a hint of that taking place in *Amoeba proteus* where the spore spends time within the parent cell before parting from it.

In the course of evolution and pursuit of efficiency, 'biological rhythm' behaviour became attached to a rotation between the open and the separated conditions; the combined phenomena created a more efficient 'shift' system than through rhythms alone. This has meant that periods of sleep became universal throughout animal life, but self-containment was also enlisted when exceptional internal physiological activity had to take place. It is apparent in the lives of butterflies and moths. During the self-contained egg stage, a butterfly changes from a single cell to a fully functioning caterpillar; in the equally self-contained pupal stage it matures from a caterpillar to a fully functioning adult.

In the course of evolution, the **rotating behavioural condition** became so important that it acquired its own **autonomic, two-part nervous system**: (a) the **sympathetic** orchestrates openness to the external environment whilst (b) the **parasympathetic** diminishes it.

From Wikipedia: The sympathetic nervous system is often considered the 'fight or flight' system, while the parasympathetic nervous system has been labelled the 'rest and digest' or 'feed and breed' system.[17]

A more modern characterization – *that correlates closely with this concept* – is that the sympathetic nervous system is a 'quick response

---

[17] https://en.wikipedia.org/wiki/Sympathetic_nervous_system,
https://en.wikipedia.org/wiki/Parasympathetic_nervous_system.

mobilizing system' and the parasympathetic is a 'more slowly activated dampening system'.

Placed in a behavioural context, we impose on the environment in the apertic mode. In the recedic the process is reversed; the external environment dictates how we act.

Our personalities are also shaped by the two poles: one tending to the expansive, 'extrovert', and the other self-contained, 'introvert'. But both personalities adjust – **constantly adapt** – their response according to social circumstances.

We change our attitude half-consciously during the day as we move from home to being recedic at school or work, then we turn to being apertic, expansive in play, in the pub or in other social venues. In effect, we morph into different personalities, shaped by the social environment we choose to be in.

Actors are admired for practising morphological skills but that admiration does not necessarily follow for ordinary acquaintances. Anthony Powell describes the attribute in one of his characters, Odo Stevens,[18] in 'The Dance to the Music of Time' series:

> 'At different times he would vary the line he took, rough diamond, ambitious young provincial salesman, journalist on the make, soldier of fortune, professional womanizer. Those were just a few of them all played with a lightness of touch. Stevens was certainly well aware, too, of possibility to charm by sheer lack of any too exact a definition of personality or background.'

There is an interesting species that vividly reflects the contrasting natures. Garter snakes have two forms, having either striped or spotted markings. Both live in the same environment. Spotted forms blend into the background better than striped snakes but stripes make it harder to judge the speed of the snake in motion.

---

[18] Powell, Anthony, *The Soldier's Art* (William Heinemann Ltd, 1966).

When approached, spotted garter snakes usually freeze while snakes of the striped morph move rapidly away.[19]

Just as motility is exercised in different degrees and systems, from running a marathon to vascular circulation, deployment of attitude can be consciously exercised. We can be open and engaging to someone we have never met – if they arrive with someone we know. We will distance ourselves, separate, from a waiter when we want to complain about the food.

Our physiology, behaviour and personality rotate through two poles, either a self-containing (recedic) mode or expansive (apertic), outgoing mode. Voluntarily used when we adapt to current circumstances, involuntarily intruded in sleep, in involuntary recedic and apertic moods.

6. SYNCHRONY WITH OTHERS

Microscopic life arose approximately 2.5 billion years ago when the Earth, already one billion years old, was still a very unsettled environment. If micro-organisms had not been able to rotate into separated spores, it is unlikely that they would have survived. However, recurrent separation had consequences: it prevented connection with anything else in the environment, including other cells.

Approximately 600 million years ago, a benign period followed a prolonged cold interval known as 'Snowball Earth'. Of relevance for the current work is that the change of climate inadvertently reduced the stimulus, the need to spend as much time in the separated state. Two cells could remain in contact for long periods and if they were similar[20] their rhythms of oscillation would coincide, gain momentum and reinforce vital physiology. Once it had arisen, the evolutionary change that generated a more robust physiology was enhanced like wildfire and a flood of multicellular forms erupted.

---

[19] Campbell, Neil A., *Biology* (The Benjamin Cummings Pub. Co. Inc., 4th edition, 1996) p 426.

[20] Identical oscillation was not essential: when two oscillating bodies are in contact their oscillations move to coincide.

The essential component of multicellular life was 'synchrony' of oscillation between cells in contact with each other, which brought synchrony of physiology, perception and response to events. Unconscious physical synchrony occurs in unusual human situations; one example is that the cardiac rhythms of singers can synchronize in choirs. The phenomenon of having the same perception of, and response to, the environment first occurs between mother and child. It becomes most compelling and addictive between partners 'in love'. When opportunity to experience synchrony is lost, as in widowhood, our resilience and our ability to maintain good health is diminished.

Human attachments reflect different qualities and levels of synchrony. The most important component is a unified perception of the hospitable/inhospitable state of the environment with the most appropriate, i.e. open or distancing, response. Reassuring to the newborn, it enhances well-being throughout life.

7. HIERARCHICAL POSITIONING

Every unicellular organism forms a decision on the quality of change in the environment and determines response for itself. On most occasions, cells adjacent to each other in a small multicellular organism would make the same decision and respond in the same way. However, once thousands of cells congregated together as a multicellular organism it became possible for cells at some distance from each other to differ in assessing change and determining upon the most appropriate reaction. Differing decisions would end in disintegration. It was a danger that could only be avoided by allowing one group of cells to decide upon the condition of the environment, determine a response and impose it upon the rest; in other words, a hierarchical organization. The group of dominant cells evolved into the brain and nervous system.

Imposing a perception of the environment and form of response on all other cells also carried a responsibility to make accurate decisions on the nature of change and 'best' reaction, making the neurological or behavioural system ultimately responsible for the well-being of all cells, for survival. Such a system must include feedback from tissues and organs of physiological stability. When instability occurs, e.g. through infection, the feedback will be that the Central Nervous System is not fulfilling its purpose and it will be stimulated to find strategies to cope, such as raising the body temperature to hinder pathogens.

This system is replicated in human societies where those who are hierarchically responsible for a group try to restore order when it has been lost.

In this concept, hierarchical positioning is considered an elemental behaviour.[21] We have a compulsion to place people, events and objects in a two-part hierarchy. Film stars, football players and friends are either awesome or 'past it'. Meals are delicious or mediocre. Plays, books, concerts are fantastic or not worthwhile. The second best is little regarded.

When an individual holds an unusually elevated position there is a race to duplicate their appearance, to identify with the 'star', and for some a compulsion to associate with them. Football clubs make huge profits by selling shirts with the number and name of the team's most successful players to their fans.

Hierarchy permeates and distorts our communication. When we think that one aspect of a communication is more important, we emphasize it and give a different interpretation to that which was originally passed to us. Manufacturers use the authoritarian power of labels to promote their products.[22]

Hierarchies act simultaneously, like the pecking order amongst chickens. We are hierarchically in charge of a car but, if we are wise,

---

[21] Nomadic tribes are an exception: they eschew hierarchies and withdraw from individuals who seek to impose authority. In their communities, emphasis on one elemental behaviour, motility, has diminished the need to establish hierarchy.

[22] In an experiment by Professor Regan, reported on 23 April 2009 on BBC 2, she demonstrated that branded painkillers brought more relief than identical generic products. (In effect, the brand names carried a visible authority that the tablets would diminish the subject's pain.)

we submit to the traffic lights. Domination is more easily accepted if we have someone else to dominate. In the animal world, collie dogs respond to the slightest command from the shepherd but enjoy controlling the herd of sheep. A pernicious hierarchy often occurs in prisons whilst those with the greatest mobility and freedom, the nomads of the steppes, actively reject hierarchy.

In many successful marriages an alternating balance is achieved, with one partner making decisions in one area of the couple's lives whilst the other directs elsewhere. However, many women suffer from 'control freaks', from partners who have little authority elsewhere and are addicted to hierarchical dominance at home.

The healthy hierarchical position is being in control of one's life, having the freedom to go where we wish and to choose a pattern of life that we are at ease with. However, the environment is impaired for everyone when an individual who is addicted to perceiving themselves as 'superior' constantly seeks to demonstrate to him or herself that they are in control of whatever happens. In that self-deception, city drivers of four-wheel-drive vehicles are four times more likely than drivers of other cars to use hand-held mobile phones and they are less likely to comply with the law on seat belts.[23] Accepting a hierarchy may be lifesaving or disastrous: health, for example, can be restored by submitting to medical advice but popular submission to Adolf Hitler was catastrophic for Europe.[24]

A balanced hierarchical condition is beneficial; unrelieved abasement can cause depression, and it is easy to see that high political status and recognition as a celebrity both become addictive, i.e. have momentum. Professor Makiko Yamada and colleagues at the National Institute of Radiological Sciences labelled the susceptibility of an individual to believe that they are above others the

---

[23] Walker, Lesley et al., 'Unsafe driving behaviour and four wheel drive vehicles: observational study', BMJ, Vol 333, 8 July 2006, pp 71–74.

[24] 'We maintain our integrity only by withstanding other people's controlling behaviour.' Dominants coerce, blackmail others into compliance. Forward, Susan, 'Emotional Blackmail', in Butler-Bowdon, Tom, ed., *50 Psychology Classics* (Nicholas Brealey Publishing, 2012) p 94.

'superiority illusion' and found that it was associated with high levels of dopamine in the brain.[25]

Alternatively, the acceptance of hierarchical direction can be attractive because it relieves us of responsibility for decisions, ultimately diminishing the need to choose which personality state or attitude to be in.[26]

We have a predisposition to categorize ourselves, the social and material environment in hierarchical form.

SUMMARY

The elemental behaviours can function:

a) Completely unconsciously. We are unaware of oscillation and many of the circadian rhythms that take place within us.

b) We can consciously recognize some involuntary behaviours such as respiration, sleep and cyclical depression.

c) A behaviour can be forced upon us by a need to separate from intolerable circumstances when we cannot walk away, e.g. uncontrollably falling asleep (i.e. separating from the environment) in the middle of a battle.

d) We can make conscious choices to move, to shape our attitude, to enter into synchrony, to submit or take charge of events (i.e. hierarchically take control).

It is worth noticing that we project characteristics of elemental behaviours onto the external environment without justification. For

---

[25] '...that they are more intelligent and have a greater number of desirable personality traits with a higher cognitive ability than the average person.' Yamada M., et al., 'Superiority illusion arises from resting-state brain networks modulated by dopamine', *Proceedings of the National Academy of Sciences of the United States of America*, 12 Mar 2013, 110(11):4363-4367. doi: 10.1073/pnas.1221681110.

[26] Eric Hoffer summarized this as, 'People allow themselves to be swept up in larger causes in order to be freed of responsibility for their lives and to escape the banality or misery of the present.' Hoffer, Eric, 'The True Believer', in Butler-Bowdon, Tom, ed., *50 Psychology Classics* (Nicholas Brealey Publishing, 2012) p 152.

example, environments that coincide with self-containment – such as night-time and sleep – persuade us that the night is likely to be inhospitable. Giving high hierarchical status to events such as opera and objects like jewellery makes it more likely that we will spend money to 'submit' to them.

* * *

The elemental behaviours also generate subsystems that can become independent. Cardiac pulsation, normally 'managed' by the autonomic nervous system, is capable of independent function. Similarly, sleep and depressed mood, normally subject to rhythmical physiological 'management', develop independent cycles in Kleine-Levin Syndrome.[27]

The need to exercise all behavioural resources also means that both poles of a behavioural trait have to be occasionally expressed: 'Going green may make you mean,' Kate Connolly reported.[28] 'When people feel they have been morally virtuous [self-inhibiting or recedic] ... it leads to ... "the licensing [of] selfish [apertic] and morally questionable behaviour".' In other words, submitting to ethical expectations will alternate with assertiveness and selfishness in a different area.

The reverse also holds: students who binge drink are more likely than others to join the United States military... and as binge

---

[27] From Wikipedia: 'Kleine-Levin Syndrome (KLS), also known as "Sleeping Beauty syndrome", is a rare sleep disorder characterized by persistent episodic hypersomnia and cognitive or mood changes. Many patients also experience hyperphagia, hypersexuality and other symptoms. Patients generally experience recurrent episodes of the condition for more than a decade. Individual episodes generally last more than a week but less than a month. The condition greatly affects the personal, professional, and social lives of sufferers, but symptoms spontaneously resolve and seldom cause permanent issues. The severity of symptoms and the course of the disease vary between sufferers. Patients commonly have about 20 episodes over about a decade. Several months generally elapse between episodes. The onset of the condition usually follows a viral infection.' https://en.wikipedia.org/wiki/Kleine–Levin_syndrome

[28] Guardian.co.uk, 15 March 2010, from work by Nina Mazar and Chen-Bo Zhong, 'Do green products make us better people?', *Psychological Science*, April 2010, pp 494–498.

drinking increased so did the propensity to join the military.[29] Undisciplined youths, used to indulging themselves, choose at one point to 'submit' to discipline, to be controlled.

In summary, seven elemental behaviours have been proposed. They reinforce the physiology of microscopic life and *when moderately exercised, facilitate human health.*

---

[29] *Military Medicine* 2013, 178:37-42, reported in *The Week.*

CHAPTER 6

FOOD, SEX AND APPETITE

It will not have escaped notice that two human preoccupations, sexual intercourse and eating, have not been considered elemental behaviours.

In the simplest possible proposition, organic particles adhere to and are absorbed by micro-organisms and many cells (such as our white blood corpuscles) very easily. Those micro-organisms that ingested and metabolized the adherent particles gained significant advantage.

In another progression, contact with an identical individual with similar oscillation could progress to merging and sexual reproduction.

As one behaviour is advantageous to the individual and the other to perpetuation of the species, natural selection appears to have added appetite to the two advantageous behaviours. In effect, the powerful oscillation and accompanying biochemical changes that are attached to particularly hospitable events have been energetically applied to ingestion and sexual reproduction.

When a new evolutionary strategy arises, (i) it may not necessarily be accurately targeted, (ii) it becomes available to other traits and (iii) it can have reverse application.

i)   I was once asked to see a fourteen-year-old boy who persisted in approaching elderly ladies and sexually harassing them. It was subsequently revealed that he had been seduced by an elderly lady into his first sexual experience and ejaculation. 'Added appetite' can take equally compulsive but less damaging forms in fetishism.

ii) Positive appetite attraction can be applied to engaging habits such as collecting antiques, keeping pets, creating art, etc.

iii) At the opposite pole, negative rejection of objects, animals and circumstances such as enclosed spaces can become appetite-enhanced phobias. Nausea and vomiting that have occurred by chance with a particular food can lead to long-lasting disgust.

In short, unlike the elemental behaviours, 'added appetite' is an unpredictable stimulus, a 'wild card'.

CHAPTER 7

BEHAVIOURAL PROPRIOCEPTION

MONITORING ONE'S OWN EMOTIONS

A vital part of the neuromuscular system is the proprioceptive[1] subsystem that unconsciously monitors and adjusts muscles and joints to preserve our upright condition. It enables the brain to 'know' the position we are in at any time: the point that any new activity has to start from. If I want a drink and am lying down, I need to undertake quite different movements to those that I would carry out if I was sitting. Awareness (largely subconscious) of what direction is up and what is down in the environment and my starting point are critical to undertaking any task.

The resource has its own cerebral organ, the cerebellar lobes. The information and myriad slight adjustments are facilitated through its own tracts, which have the fastest transmission rates of the nervous system. My contention is that without an equivalent behavioural proprioception, awareness of our behavioural condition as well as our physical position, our behaviour will be badly managed. The

---

[1] Wikipedia: 'Proprioception is the sense of the relative position of neighbouring parts of the body and strength of effort being employed in movement... It is distinguished from exteroception, by which one perceives the outside world, and interoception, by which one perceives pain, hunger, etc., and the movement of internal organs. The brain integrates information from proprioception and from the vestibular system into its overall sense of body position, movement, and acceleration.' https://en.wikipedia.org/wiki/Proprioception

crucial sense is one of being aware of which behavioural mode, apertic or recedic, we are in. The physical proprioceptive system is exercised early in life as babies learn how to hold and pass an object from one hand to another. Behavioural proprioception is more gradually established from experiences throughout childhood.

Recent research by Ilaria Carta and others suggests that the cerebellum has a role in the expression of behaviour: 'To perform its functions the cerebellum is believed to integrate these diverse inputs to provide the rest of the brain with predictions required for optimal behaviour.'[2] In other words, new research would seem to confirm that the cerebellar system may facilitate behavioural as well as physical proprioception.

Talented authors can recognize the dynamic of a behavioural phenomenon when others have failed to do so. John Bew, in his biography of Clement Attlee,[3] writes, 'What distinguished him from the pack was not ambition, though he was not without this – so much as a self-awareness lacking in many of his peers.' The skill can be compared to a chess player who knows without thinking about it that he/she is behaving most wisely in a recedic mode to safeguard the king, or alternatively, behaving in an apertic mode to checkmate an opponent.

Behavioural proprioception, like physical proprioception, has little consciousness so is easily ignored when we are distracted by external events, such as when we are sexually attracted. It means that just when we need to be aware of being apertic, possibly too expansive, we fail to recognize it.

Behavioural proprioception is acutely important to another human behaviour, alternation.

---

[2] Carta, I. et al., 'Cerebellar modulation of the reward circuitry and social behavior', published in *Science* Vol 363 issue 6424, 18 Jan 2019.

[3] Bew, John, *Citizen Clem: A Biography of Attlee* (Riverrun, 2017) p 200.

ALTERNATION

There are two forms of synchrony: one where perceptions and responses are in close coordination and another where an assertive peak of one individual (apogee) matches the trough (nadir) of another. It is a universal experience as we alternate in conversation with one individual being recedic as the other expansively speaks. The alternation can be more invigorating than quiet synchrony where apogees and nadirs correlate, but for conversation to be satisfying to both participants there needs to be balance of both volume and period of intrusion by the 'apogee' participant in his or her turn.

The habit of alternation in human society may be used in extraordinary circumstances. Police and other negotiators are taught the process without knowing why it succeeds.

Behavioural proprioception contributes to emotional intelligence and alternation to coexistence.

CHAPTER 8

INTELLIGENCE

The first characteristic of change that registers is the volume of change. Extreme volume of change such as an earthquake can occur in the natural environment. The equivalent in the social environment is a close family member being killed in front of one. Both cause a reflex-like drive to separate from the event. If there is no opportunity to move away to another environment we become immobile, paralysed.

If the 'volume' of change has not provoked a reflex response it is instantly qualified as hospitable or inhospitable; in this concept, intelligence is built upon that duopoly.

When an environment is challenging, survival depends upon deciding whether an event is hospitable or inhospitable as quickly as possible. Metaphorically, when a warrior is challenged he has to immediately decide whether his opponent is weaker (hospitable) or stronger (inhospitable) than he is, whether to take up his sword or his shield. Once the sword or shield is decided upon, perception and attitude have momentum and only change if circumstances alter dramatically or the momentum wears off.

When the environment is consistently benign, both perceptions and responses become less polarized. A warrior will be able to observe others' both aggressive (apertic) and weaker (recedic) aspects and discover more about an individual than from polarized conclusions driven by the need to survive. When there is no need to practise with swords and shields other activities can take place and the weapons be used as tools. In short, the **recedic position and the**

apertic position can be used together to assess and respond to unthreatening events.

It may be difficult to understand why the combination can lead to greater intelligence. Better intelligence arises from having as much knowledge as possible immediately available. A second more contemporary metaphor may help.

Imagine travelling from a London terminus to one's own home town. There are two trains from different platforms, one a slow train stopping at several stations and ending up at a station closest to home; it is cheaper and very reliable. There is a fast train, on another platform, that is leaving shortly and will arrive at a different station slightly further away from one's home, needing a short taxi ride.

In a recedic mood I choose the slow, reliable train; in an apertic mood I pay more and choose the fast train as I would like to arrive home as early as possible.

However, if both trains can be accessed from either side of one platform I am able to see advantages and disadvantages that I might otherwise have missed, such as a friend I want to see getting on the other train or that they are already standing on the train I was going to get on whilst the other is uncrowded. It is only by accessing change in the environment from the simultaneous platform, holding both points of view, that I am able to make the most advantageous choice.

It is very difficult to retain divergent perceptions at the same time but the success it brought when it was achieved perpetuated the ability.

A new intellectual ability was established when a benign climate made it possible to assess events and respond from the apertic and recedic 'platforms' simultaneously.

The process was carried further through millennia of primate evolution.

CHAPTER 9

PRIMATE EVOLUTION

PRIMATES

There will have been many complex, subtle steps in the evolution of intelligence and a new direction for hominids. Behavioural scientists and psychiatrists will say that any attempt to condense such events into a few pages is facile. Charles Darwin dedicated his life and assembled an immense quantity of evidence to establish the 'Origin of Species'. I have neither the time, as an octogenarian, nor the resources to carry out a similar exercise. I have limited myself to bringing significant events and phenomena into a logical progression.

Between five and two million years ago, the climate in East Africa passed through very benign periods. Food became so abundant that it diminished the challenge to survive, facilitating social cohesion and intelligence, which reduced the challenge even more. Whenever stimulus is diminished, degeneration beckons and, in this case, threatened the viability of the great ape family.

Almost by chance, new social patterns and behaviours evolved and sparked a faint sense of self-esteem, a slight but enjoyable feeling, sufficiently pleasing to make individuals want to relive it. The new reward for successful behaviour was intensified, arrested degeneration and was extended in hominids to become a new 'operating' system.

A benign climate moderated reflex-like responses and allowed differing perceptions to be held together – a first step to greater intellectual ability. A cycle followed: the combination of a benign environment and greater intelligence diminished the challenge to survive. A lack of challenges diminished the dominant male's role in leading activity; it allowed the community to pay attention to and copy skills of any member who displayed them. Any intelligent member could lead the group in an activity. The development continued with more and more success, leading to survival becoming less and less challenging. Absence of challenge, of purpose, ultimately threatens degeneration (c.f. optic lobes in blind crustaceans, page 18), which could only be averted by changing the 'operating system' or purpose.

Before moving to the new operating system, 'emotional' intelligence needs clarification.

There are two intellectual streams: (i) creating and using tools and (ii) emotional intelligence, 'knowing oneself' and 'knowing others'. The latter can be more rewarding.

EMOTIONAL INTELLIGENCE

Social or emotional intelligence has two parts.

> From Wikipedia: **Social intelligence**, the capacity to know oneself and to know others, is as inalienable a part of the human condition as is the capacity to know objects or sounds, and it deserves to be investigated no less than the other 'less charged' forms.[1]

In short, behavioural proprioception, monitoring one's own emotions, is one half of social or emotional intelligence; the other half is being able to 'read' another's emotional responses.

---

[1] https://en.wikipedia.org/wiki/Social_intelligence

Emotions are disclosed in:

- Facial expression
- Facial colour
- Posture or body language
- Timbre of voice
- And an olfactory element we may not consciously register.

Biologists often label the emotions that we show as 'signals'. That is misleading; signals are consciously expressed and intentionally conveyed. The above phenomena are reflex-like and involuntarily declare how events have been experienced.

Some individuals, such as successful poker players, manage to conceal their responses. Children who have been treated cruelly and suffered more when they have shown emotion also learn to suppress it. Psychopaths learn to flag up emotions they do not actually feel. Actors find it possible to display a false emotion by imagining an appropriate event. Different races and genders may vary in the quality and degree of reflex expression due to cultural factors.[2]

Those circumstances apart, and unlike emotions conveyed by artificial language, the involuntary phenomena are usually honest revelations of how we feel and they are difficult to suppress:

a) Facial expression. We have a large number of small facial muscles that show fine degrees of emotion. Combinations of eyes, eyebrow, lips, nose and cheek movements declare both the nature and degree of response.

b) Facial colour. Whilst revising this work the digital version of *The Times* (of 20 March 2018) reported the following:

---

[2] Bond, Michael Harris, 'Emotions and their expression in Chinese culture', *Journal of Nonverbal Behavior*, 17(4) December 1993, pp 245–262. Human Sciences Press Inc. 'What differs in Chinese culture is the lower frequency, intensity and duration with which emotions are typically experienced… evidence suggests that the expression of emotion is carefully regulated out of concern for its capacity to disrupt group harmony and status hierarchies.'

'We are used to the idea that skin colouration can convey extreme emotion but a recent study has shown that it is an effective *signal*[3] [my emphasis] of all the moods in between too. Most people think they can spot what people are feeling by looking at their facial muscles but it turns out that we can do almost as well just by looking at their cheeks. The research was carried out by Alex Martinez from the Ohio State University. For his study, published in the *Proceedings of the National Academy of Sciences*, he wanted to see if these blood vessels served a purpose by *signalling* emotion [my emphasis]. He and his colleagues trained a computer to spot subtle differences of colour in faces expressing different emotions. More than 80 per cent of the time people were able to identify the one that matched the emotion. He said that this showed just how crucial picking up on subtle social cues must be for humans. It is very important for us to know how others are feeling.'

c) Body postures. Both sitting and standing postures indicate emotions. A person sitting to the back of their chair, leaning forward with their head nodding along with the discussion, implies that they are open, relaxed and generally ready to listen. On the other hand, a person who has their legs and arms crossed with the foot kicking slightly implies that they are feeling impatient and emotionally detached from the discussion.

d) Timbre of voice. This is perhaps the easiest to imitate so actors use it frequently to try to convey emotion.

We can be ill at ease when engaged in conversation and may be aware or unaware of exhibiting our reflex emotional responses. If we are embarrassed, for example, we blush, and whether we are conscious of blushing will depend on how engaged we happen to be.

---

[3] Involuntary reflex responses.

Registering our own and recognizing emotional responses in others is a significant attribute. If those we are in conversation with show no reflex emotions, either through intentional control or through a relative absence of the attribute, we become ill at ease. It is also important to recognize any dichotomy of reflex emotions, conflicting responses in those we engage with. A lack of wrinkles around the eyes, for example, suggests a fake, sham smile; it means only superficial concurrence with what has been said.

Television editors are alert to actions that indicate difference with what is being said and direct the camera to an interviewee's clutched fingers or feet tapping away. Honest emotions visible to others are essential to trust and cooperation.

Without artificial language, emotional reflex knowledge must be more important for chimpanzees than it is for us. Behaviourists have discovered that chimpanzees have a long childhood and consider its advantages. They focus upon the opportunities to learn from others to identify the most nutritious food and how it can be obtained. Such lessons could be learnt in passing through the seasons for two years, but it takes much longer to recognize the many social cues, where and when they occur and how best to respond to them. Social learning is essential for personal security and important for the harmony of the whole group.

PRIMATE LIFE

Both social and physical skills increased in primates; they exercised and extended intelligence and ultimately made survival easier, less challenging and threatened degeneration of the skills used in surviving. A new drive, a new purpose, gradually arose: pursuing and gaining self-esteem. Self-esteem could be acquired through settling differences, engaging in skills that are copied, but also in competitive and clandestine behaviour, cheating and manipulating others.

During the course of evolution primates separated into different branches. Hominids did not evolve from bonobos but from a branch that divided slightly earlier. It is, however, assumed in this work that the earliest steps to intelligence and a new 'operating system' evolved similarly in both species but progressed further in hominids.

As primates, and particularly chimpanzees, evolved, they acquired acute awareness of how other members of the group were feeling through reflex emotions. It could be compared to cellular oscillatory synchrony that facilitated multicellular life. It enabled the tribe to act as one but with the intellectual resources of many whenever predators threatened.

Several stages had to take place before unity could be attained:

1. A benign climatic environment was vital: 'In a year of poor harvest the chimpanzees become less sociable.'[4]
2. One early, necessary step was to be able to register the emotions and actions of more than one other individual at the same time. The more primitive primates, lemurs, could only act dyadically, that is, only relate to one other at a time.[5]
3. With evolution, female hamadryas baboons 'expertly exploited the properties of adult males in threatening other females from a protected and powerful position'. In short, they were able to triadically register the actions and emotions of 'adult male' and 'other female' and manipulate them simultaneously.[6]

    Minimal conflict between individuals was essential. It could not be achieved in baboons because 'both sexes frequently become involved in the maintenance of a prolonged state of

---

[4] Wrangham, R. W., 'Behavioural ecology of chimpanzees in Gombe National Park, Tanzania'. Unpublished PhD thesis (1975), University of Cambridge, quoted by Nicholas K. Humphrey in *Machiavellian Intelligence* (Clarendon Press Oxford, 1988).
[5] Jolly, A., *The Evolution of Primate Behavior* (Macmillan, 2nd edition, 1985) quoted by Whiten and Byrne, ibid. p 8.
[6] Kummer, F. B. M. (1967), recorded in Harcourt, A. H. and de Waal, F. B. M. (eds), *Coalitions and Alliances in Humans and Other Animals* (OUP, 1992). Quoted by Byrne and Whiten, *Machiavellian Intelligence II* (Cambridge University Press, 1997) p 4.

unresolved conflict'.[7] Every member of the tribe needed to be working to the same script, akin to the unity of a choir that induces synchronous cardiac pulsation. (Synchrony with others, page 31.)

4. Hierarchy (dominant male authority) had to be attenuated so that any member of the tribe could decide whether a change was hospitable/inhospitable. It is evident in the advanced bonobos: 'The species is best characterized as female-centred and egalitarian and as one that substitutes sex for aggression. Whereas in most other species, sexual behaviour is a fairly distinct category, in the bonobo it is part and parcel of social relations – and not just between males and females.'[8]

5. There is a need to be cooperative even in situations that militate against sharing. 'When presented with a task of retrieving food that was difficult to monopolize (keep to oneself), bonobos and chimpanzees were equally cooperative. However, when the food reward was highly monopolizable, bonobos were more successful than chimpanzees at cooperating to retrieve it.'[9]

In summary, bonobos achieved a high degree of synchrony through reflex expression of emotions and cooperative behaviour. They also achieved intellectual prowess that puzzled observers:

i) 'What are primates doing with their superior intelligence?'[10]

ii) 'Nature is surely at least as careful an economist as Henry Ford. It is not her habit to tolerate needless extravagance in the animals on her production lines: superfluous capacity is trimmed back,

---

[7] Chance, M. R. A. and Mead, A. P. 'Social behaviour and primate evolution', Symposia of the Society of Experimental Biology Evolution 7 (1953) pp 395–439. Quoted by Whiten and Byrne, *Machiavellian Intelligence II* (Cambridge University Press, 1997) p 11.

[8] De Waal, Frans B. M., 'Bonobo Sex and Society', *Scientific American*, 1 Jun 2006.

[9] Hare, Brian et al., 'Tolerance allows bonobos to outperform chimpanzees on a cooperative task', *Journal of Current Biology*, Vol 17, issue 7, pp 619–623, 3 April 2007.

[10] Whiten and Byrne, *Machiavellian Intelligence*, (Clarendon Press, 1988) p 6.

new capacity only added as and when it is needed. We do not expect, therefore, to find that animals present abilities which far exceed the demands that natural living makes on them.'[11]

iii) N. K. Humphrey struggles to give reason for the increased intelligence:

> 'I have suggested that the life of the great apes and man may not require much in the way of practical invention but it does depend critically on the possession of wide factual knowledge of practical technique and the nature of the material and social habitat. Such knowledge can only be acquired in the context of a social community – a community which provides both a medium for the cultural transmission of information and a protective environment in which the individual learning can occur.'

But to correlate with the competitive survival principle, Humphrey puts the cart before the horse: 'I propose that the chief role of creative intellect is to hold society together.'[12]

Put the other way around, in the context of this work, social living exercises intelligence – leading to its growth beyond facilitating survival.

Possibly the most important phenomenon in relation to this concept is a study by Povinelli in 1992. A two-player cooperative task is tested with both rhesus monkeys and chimpanzees.[13] It is a striking example of instant mode rotation, the genesis of intelligence:

> 'One player can see which handle will provide both with food rewards but not operate the handle; the other cannot see which to pull but can operate both handles. Both species

---

[11] Humphrey, Nicholas K., *Machiavellian Intelligence* (Clarendon Press, 1988) p 22.

[12] Ibid., p 18.

[13] 'Comprehension of role reversal in chimpanzees: evidence of empathy?', Povinelli, D. J. et al. (1992), *Animal Behaviour*, 43(4), pp 633–640.

learn either role in the task. However, when an individual
that has learnt one role is placed in the other the results are
quite different. Monkeys have to learn the whole task again
while the chimpanzee is able to assume the other role without
retraining. The result shows understanding of the physical
cause and effect logic of the cooperative task but whether this
requires an understanding of the mental states of the other
individual is less definite.'

In short, one directs apertically and the other acts recedically. Each
rotates without hesitation to the alternate role.

Primates evolved through moving from dyadic to triadic awareness and became able to:

i)   register contrasting states: dominance in an adult male and
     self-containing in another female;
ii) act with opposite responses: recedic to the male, apertic upon
     the female;
iii) create change by manipulating the adult male – all simultaneously.

The loss of stimulation by unity and growth of intelligence was
recognized by N. K. Humphrey:[14]

> 'The great apes, demonstrably the most intellectually gifted
> of all animals, seem on the whole to lead comparatively
> undemanding lives, less demanding not only than those of
> lower primates but also many non-primate species.'

Humphrey's observation and evidence in Povinelli's experiment
of greater ability than is necessary in their natural circumstances
supports the contention that the challenge to survive no longer fully

---

[14] Quoted in Whiten and Byrne, *Machiavellian Intelligence* (Clarendon Press, 1988)
p 17.

exercised the advanced primates and an alternative purpose was vital. In this concept, it was found in a drive for self-satisfaction, for self-esteem. The first signs of it developing can be discerned in captive chimpanzees:

1. 'Figan had not only refrained from instantly gratifying his desire but had gone away so that he could not give the game away by looking at the banana.'[15]
2. 'They hide themselves and hide objects.' [to deceive others][16]
3. 'Kanzi takes great delight in flaunting his ability to pick and eat mushrooms without being detected.'[17]
4. 'Much of the tactical deception in primates is concerned with the manipulation of the attention of other individuals.'[18]

---

[15] Goodall. J, *In the Shadow of Man* (Collins, 1971) quoted in Humphrey, Nicholas K., *Machiavellian Intelligence* (Clarendon Press, 1988) p 219.

[16] Savage-Rumbaugh, Sue and MacDonald, Kelly, 'Deception and social manipulation in symbol-using apes' quoted in *Machiavellian Intelligence* (Clarendon Press, 1988) p 231.

[17] Ibid., p 230.

[18] Humphrey, Nicholas K., *Machiavellian Intelligence* (Clarendon Press, 1988) p 212.

CHAPTER 10

NEW 'OPERATING SYSTEM'

The pursuit of self-esteem places a premium on gaining social respect and the ability to manipulate tools and natural materials.

No one, as far as I am aware, has suggested a site in the brain for the biological, survival determination of human behaviour or how it could bring to bear an influence on our behaviour.

In contrast, both the mechanism and site for the function of self-esteem can be found through the work of A. R. Liss: 'Executive functions (collectively referred to as executive function and cognitive control) are a set of cognitive processes that are necessary for the cognitive control of behaviour: selecting and successfully monitoring behaviours that facilitate the attainment of chosen goals.'[1]

And later in the work: 'The prefrontal cortex is necessary but not solely sufficient for executive functions; for example, the caudate nucleus and subthalamic nucleus also have a role in mediating inhibitory control.'

In short, the executive functions that determine our behaviour are primarily found in the prefrontal area of the frontal lobes.

Injury and dysfunction of the frontal lobes also indicate that self-awareness and self-esteem are located at that site. It was first noted in an historically famous case: Phineas P. Gage (1823–1860)

---

[1] Lezak, M.D. (1989). 'Assessment of psychosocial dysfunctions resulting from head trauma', originally in *Assessment of the behavioural consequences of head trauma* (pp 113–143). New York: Alan R. Liss.

was an American railroad construction foreman remembered for
his improbable survival of an accident in which a large iron rod
was driven completely through his head, destroying much of his
brain's left frontal lobe, and for that injury's reported effects on his
personality and behaviour over the remaining twelve years of his life
– effects sufficiently profound (for a time at least) that friends saw
him as 'no longer Gage'.[2]

Medical injury of the frontal lobes was carried out in the 1940s
and 1950s as a treatment for overwhelming, resistant anxiety and
other conditions:

> From Wikipedia: A **lobotomy**, or leucotomy, is a form of
> psychosurgery, a neurosurgical treatment of a mental disorder
> that involves severing connections in the brain's prefrontal
> cortex. Most of the connections to and from the prefrontal
> cortex, the anterior part of the frontal lobes of the brain are
> severed. It was used for psychiatric and occasionally other
> conditions as a mainstream procedure in some Western
> countries for more than two decades…
>
> … The lobotomy procedure could have severe negative
> effects on a patient's personality and ability to function
> independently. Lobotomy patients often show a marked reduction
> in initiative and inhibition.[3]

MEDICAL DISORDER

Those affected by a rare clinical condition, Cotard's syndrome,
believe that they are dead, that they no longer exist. Both the character of the condition and the associated physiological changes
indicate that the sense of self is located in the frontal lobes.

---

[2] https://en.wikipedia.org/wiki/Phineas_Gage
[3] https://en.wikipedia.org/wiki/Lobotomy

From a *New Scientist* 'Mindscapes' column on brain science:

> 'A peek inside Graham's brain provided Zeman and
> Laureys with some explanation. They used positron
> emission tomography to monitor metabolism across his
> brain. It was the first PET scan ever taken of a person
> with Cotard's. What they found was shocking: metabolic
> activity across large areas of the frontal and parietal brain
> regions was so low that it resembled that of someone in a
> vegetative state.'[4]

EVOLUTION

In the past century, many hominid fossil skeletons have been found that show a steady increase in size of the brain, particularly of the forebrain.[5]

Frontal lobe enlargement in hominids and the drive to self-esteem that accompanied it undoubtedly brought success but also carried an Achilles' heel, a vulnerability. Striving for self-esteem places us on a knife edge that is easy to fall from on one side or the other. When our striving cannot be satisfied, when success eludes us, there is despair, depression, loss of self-respect – conditions that can be recedic. Falling on the other side can give rise to manic energy, egocentricity, preoccupation with hierarchy, greed and diminishing the value of the underprivileged to justify separating from them; apertic phenomena that are considered more valuable than maladaptive in Western society.

---

4 Thomson, Helen, 'Mindscapes: First interview with a dead man', *New Scientist*, 23 May 2013. Available online at https://www.newscientist.com/article/dn23583-mindscapes-first-interview-with-a-dead-man/
5 John Pickrell provides an informative illustration of fossil skull development in 'Timeline: Human Evolution', *New Scientist*, 4 September 2006. Available online at https://www.newscientist.com/article/dn9989-timeline-human-evolution/

Self-esteem[6] can be gathered from the respect of others for the skills that one can display *or* from success in gaining personal advantage; occasionally from both at the same time. In John le Carré's autobiographical fiction *A Perfect Spy*,[7] his politician father worked hard to help the deprived but at the same time cheated the pensioners of their savings. The behaviour also happens at an insignificant level; giving presents that have been taking up space in a cupboard or unwanted food to the food bank can be small reasons for self-congratulation.

In short, when living necessities are satisfied we are no longer preoccupied with survival. The purpose has been replaced by a barely conscious but very sensitive need for self-esteem. It is as compulsive as a cell's need to maintain its physiology. Although the combination of intelligence and search for self-esteem has enabled us to dominate the planet, it brings misery for those who cannot satisfy the compulsion and insidious addiction when it is acquired.

Unsatisfied self-esteem makes the transient pleasures of drugs, alcohol, smoking, overeating and taking risks tempting displacements. Pursuit of the emotion is most acute and most difficult to satisfy in adolescent life. When it cannot be found, adolescents punish themselves with self-harm or, worse, commit suicide. The situation is exacerbated when teenagers are flooded with images of stars and sportsmen little older than themselves who have achieved heroic status. The celebrities feel it is their role to assert that anyone can 'will' it and do the same. The celebrities are satisfying their own drive for self-esteem by implying that they only succeeded through personal behaviour, they 'willed' it. No question that they might have succeeded because they had one or more advantages: handsome appearance, better intelligence, better strength and

---

[6] I have thought about the label self-esteem for many hours. The emotion is compounded of self-esteem, pride, egocentricity and identity. It requires a new label and I have considered 'eyam' in earlier drafts. Settling on self-esteem appeared to be the closest and simplest label that others can relate to.

[7] le Carré, John, *A Perfect Spy* (Hodder and Stoughton, 1986).

coordination or just plain good luck. Their assertion that success can be 'willed' brings misery to the majority who cannot emulate their success.

The Industrial Revolution, globalization and television have made it very difficult to find ways to build self-esteem. For adults, vegetables are so cheap it is scarcely worthwhile trying to find value in gardening skills or having an allotment. Incredibly cheap clothes, worn once or twice, make dressmaking redundant.

One word describes the pursuit of self-esteem: 'meretricious'. When flourishing, it is shiny and seductive but when lost, a source of misery. The self-esteem 'operating system' is most evident when it is threatened or could be enhanced. The saying 'success has many fathers; failure is an orphan' reflects the dynamic. We always need to voice that we have played a significant part in any successful enterprise and even more quickly distance ourselves from a debacle.

We remember our social, academic and sporting successes with pleasure but the shaming memory of making a 'gaffe', of failing to appraise the social environment correctly, e.g. making a rude joke about Americans only to find that we are talking to one, can also remain with us for the rest of our lives. Throughout our adulthood, public loss of respect by ill-judged behaviour brings loss of synchrony with society and loss of hierarchical status within it.

In Western society, self-esteem has many addictive gratifications that range from winning a Nobel Prize, Olympic Gold medals, through *Games People Play*[8] to winning the monthly pub quiz. Our respect for ourselves can also be lodged in how we have acted in fulfilling the best interests of others. For many middle-aged couples, how well they have parented their children is measured by the child's social success. For Nicolas Chauvin, it was his service to Napoleon. When all enhancing opportunities are lost, the elderly advertise their years and invalids relate their disabilities. Both are excusing *themselves* for their loss of competence.

---

[8] Berne, Eric, *Games People Play* (Andre Deutsch Ltd, 1966).

Reinforcing and protecting self-esteem largely replaces biological survival as a human 'operating system' in civilized society. It carries with it a susceptibility to anxiety and dangerous self-rejection when self-esteem is unattainable or lost.

Childhood experiences can increase that susceptibility to anxiety and poor self-respect or diminish it.

CHAPTER 11

HUMAN BEHAVIOUR

The behavioural system developed from cellular physiology to maintain its steady state (homeostasis). But change was at the same time necessary to exercise the system. This contradiction recurs in our own lives. We endeavour to maintain emotional equilibrium through changing events. But we need to experience change to exercise the stabilizing faculties.

In animal life, perception of change in the environment is restricted to hospitable or inhospitable; the restoration of behavioural and emotional stability after an event is only qualified by the significance of the event and recovery time.

Restoring human equanimity is complicated by our behavioural proprioception, human intelligence and the human operating system. The complexity has been dramatically added to in recent centuries through the changing social and material conditions of the Renaissance and the Industrial Revolution, now multiplied by the digital age.

The only surprise to me is that the incidence of mental disorder is not greater than it is at present.

The most vulnerable period is childhood. The experiences that a child sustains can either engender a resilient personality capable of surviving the vicissitudes of life or burden the child with a greater susceptibility to emotional dysfunction such as personality disorder. The damaging effects of cruelty, deprivation, neglect and insecurity are well established and easily accessible online. The brain of a psychologically injured child is physically changed by such experiences, as is the child's emotional stability or psyche.[9]

There is extensive literature on the harmful experiences that children may suffer and effects that can vary with the age of the child, which makes it essential to have knowledge of how a child experiences its milieu as he/she grows up. An eight-year-old, for example, is unlikely to experience events in the same way as a baby.

It is equally essential to have good advice on parenting.

Unfortunately, there is no unified consensus on the maturation of children, and parenting advice is not as successful as one could wish. In this article by Tom Whipple in *The Times* (2 October 2017), he writes:[10]

> 'A study by Dominica Lipinski/PA, found that the more parenting manuals new mothers read, the worse they feel.
>
> Most of the more than 350 new mothers in the Welsh study had used routine-led baby manuals of one sort or another and the number of depressive symptoms they had increased with the number they had read.'

There is a need for further research into parenting but two points can be made in the context of this work.

We can all be aware of how those near to us are feeling. Research has suggested that children are more aware than adults, and I suspect that babies are most aware of all, of how those holding them, and particularly their mothers, are feeling.

The ability to enjoy and enter into eye contact and an ability to distinguish emotion in others can occur soon after birth. Research

---

[9] Psyche: the principle of mental and emotional life, conscious and unconscious – Chambers Dictionary.

[10] https://www.thetimes.co.uk/article/happy-mothers-give-baby-books-the-boot-bcfpjmwhc

underlines how sensitive babies are to the feelings of others and to separate from the inhospitable (angry eyes): 'Namely, these infants showed increased attention to happy eyes and decreased attention to angry eyes. This finding suggests that breastfeeding experience enhances prosocial tendencies in infants that are genetically at risk for autism.'[11]

The need for self-esteem of new mothers is as active as in the rest of us but that need becomes centred on their success in ensuring the contentment and well-being of their babies.

Putting these together, it is easy for a mother to lose confidence that she has fulfilled her responsibilities for caring, or to believe that her baby's crying indicates that it is not well, or to wish desperately that the baby would go to sleep. The baby senses the mother's unsettled state, which reduces the baby's security, an inhospitable condition, and a cycle of deterioration follows.

If someone else is holding the baby and fearing they are not holding it safely, or that they would sooner be doing something else, it is another inhospitable condition.

Babies have two affects – that the environment is hospitable or inhospitable, and if they consider the environment inhospitable they separate from it by crying.

* * *

A common and otherwise unexplained phenomenon, tears in our eyes, becomes rational in the context of separating from an event. When we have dust in our eyes, tears enable us to separate from the irritation. Nature economically applies the same response to separation from overwhelming events. We can cry when we enjoy extreme happiness (e.g. the return of a loved one) or when we are confronted by a grievous event such as the loss of a spouse. Newborn babies cry

---

[11] Krol, K. M., Monakhov, M., San Lai, P., Ebstein, R. P., and Grossmann, T., 'Genetic variation in CD38 and breastfeeding experience interact to impact infants' attention to social eye cues', PNAS, PLUS vol. 112 no. 39, 2015. Published online: https://www.ncbi.nlm.nih.gov/pmc/articles/PMC4593116/

frequently; adding as loud a noise as they can muster helps them to block out the uncertain environment.

Saying 'there, there' to a child, 'there is nothing to worry about', doesn't help the child, it just means that you haven't got the message that the environment is inhospitable, which stimulates the child to pronounce its verdict on the environment even more loudly.

If one can enjoy holding the baby, not saying 'there, there' but walking up and down, and find pleasure in humming a repetitive tune or nursery rhyme, the feeling that you find the world to be hospitable can gradually seep through the baby's crying and often succeed in encouraging the baby towards the same perception.

Sometimes a child can try to separate from inhospitable events in a very dramatic fashion. In 1984 a Sheffield solicitor shot his lover and her two children. Christopher,[12] aged six, survived but was blinded by a bullet that passed through his head from one side to the other.

Three weeks later I was asked to see Christopher on the adult surgical ward because he rejected treatment and persisted in trying to find chairs and any furniture that he could move to pile up around his bed.

Squeezing between upended chairs, I sat beside Christopher and said, 'I am sorry I am yet another doctor come to see you.' Christopher didn't say anything but stuck his finger in his nose and carefully rubbed the laden digit on my suit sleeve.

I said, 'If that makes you feel better, it's all right by me.'

Christopher needed to separate from everything, to know that he could achieve separation and to know that he was allowed to do it.

My advice to the staff was to place the chairs as near as possible so that he did not have to grope around to find them, and I arranged his transfer to the children's hospital as soon as I could.

---

[12] Unlike all the other cases, Christopher is his real name. Given the widespread publicity of the event, it seemed diminishing to a remarkable boy to use an alias. I have tried to locate Christopher to obtain his permission to include him in this work and regret that I have been unable to do so. I hope he will forgive me.

Happily, Christopher made a good recovery, regained his sight and left hospital after some weeks.

I had my last contact with, I believe, an aunt who fostered Christopher two years later. She told me that she had been passing the children's hospital on the upper deck of a bus with Christopher and a friend. Christopher remarked to the friend that he had been a patient in the hospital. The friend asked, 'Why was that?' Christopher casually replied, pointing to his head, 'I had a bullet through my brain, from here to here.' The friend went white.

* * *

The only action that young children can take from an overwhelming experience is to *separate* in one way or another. Christopher achieved real and symbolic separation by building a barricade around his bed. He could not separate from medical staff but chose the closest alternative, diminishing them – which he managed quite effectively.

Reprimanding him would not have helped; saying it did not matter would have taken away the value of the gesture. My need was to convey that his gesture was justified, that his inhospitable perception of his environment was entirely accurate.

There is a temptation, because our need is to bring comfort, to say things will get better; but it doesn't help. Those who are suffering want it to be recognized that the here and now is intolerable.

CHAPTER 12

CHILDHOOD MATURATION

The stages of development and growth phenomena, such as skeletal lengthening and voice deepening, vary from child to child. The process can be likened to taking a set of playing cards with the suits: spades, hearts, diamonds, clubs, in order, each suit representing a stage of development. The cards are allocated to different aspects of growth, then the pack is shuffled a *little*. The suits will largely stay in order but a few cards from each suit will be displaced – some back and some forward. In this slightly haphazard way, in many children some attributes will appear earlier than those traits usually occur in the majority and others will arrive later.

Early in the last century Jean Piaget identified three stages of childhood development:[1]

- Birth–2 years: Sensorimotor – experiencing the world through senses and actions.
- 2–6 years: Preoperational – representing things with words and images.
- 7–11 years: Concrete operational – thinking logically about concrete events and grasping concrete analogies.
- Adulthood: Formal operational thinking about hypothetical scenarios and processing abstract thoughts.

---

[1] Accessible online at www.simplypsychology.org/piaget.html

Piaget's stages relate to the development of intelligence, usually measured as IQ.

This concept has four stages where changes in the child's maturity shape its emotional intelligence and responses.

Staged development could not have arisen without precedent; the stages loosely parallel insect metamorphosis.

While the foetus is in utero there is intense physiological activity that absorbs all the available resources. It is like insect (and other) eggs, protected in the uterus from expending resources in accommodating to change in the external environment. Critical physiological developments continue in the immediate post-partum period and the newborn tries to retain a separated state:

> 'Infants are usually wide awake and active just after birth but
> for two or three weeks thereafter the most common state is
> either one of sleep with eyes closed, or a vague open-eyed
> condition in which awareness of the outside world appears
> weak and fluctuating ... Often a wakeful newborn is actively
> avoidant of experiences and this is particularly noticeable in
> noisy, highly stimulating circumstances.'[2]

---

[2] Professor C. Trevarthen in Gregory, Richard L., ed., *The Oxford Companion to the Mind* (OUP, 2nd edition, 2004) p 364.

CHAPTER 13

SENSORIMOTOR STAGE

In this work, the sensorimotor period is the second, post-foetal stage. In this stage children's 'sensorimotor' activity resembles that of insect caterpillars, moving freely, expansive upon the environment, quite unaware of threat or danger but separating in tears from what they find, or assume, is inhospitable. They are egocentric.

The need to be allowed, even facilitated, to behave in that way is illustrated by Kitty (seven months), who was referred to me by the social services. Colleagues were concerned because she showed little interest in feeding or in her surroundings. Kitty was, in effect, in a continually 'separated' state when she should have been practising Piaget's sensorimotor activity.

Kitty's mother, Mary, was sixteen when Kitty was born and she remained distracted by adolescent social life. In the 1970s and 1980s society hoped grandmothers would guide and support their daughters and grandchildren in those circumstances. But Mary's mother said, 'I had to get on with it when I had you at sixteen so you can get on with it too.'

Mary left Kitty with any acquaintance who would take her for two or three days at a time. She was passed around from one cot or pram to another like 'passing the parcel'.

Kitty's father, two years older than Mary, showed some interest in her but was preoccupied with his motorcycle. I supported the social services application to take Kitty into care but her father and his new partner, who had eleven- and twelve-year-old daughters, opposed the decision and requested that Kitty be placed with them.

I advised the court that Kitty was already disordered by her experiences and needed better than average parenting to help her to recover. The High Court judge opined that my evidence, based on psychiatric findings, had no scientific basis and gave Kitty into the care of her father.

I was asked to see Kitty again three months later. She sat listlessly in a corner of the living room because she was not allowed to move beyond a chalk line drawn across the floor. She had not grown.

After appeal by social services and return to court she was taken into care – *the point of this history is the nature and success of the understanding that she had from a devoted foster mother.*

In foster care Kitty received a lot of affection, had another infant with her and spent her days in a room that resembled a big playpen. There was nothing that she had to be careful about, no ornaments that might break, no television or record player that she was told not to touch; a floor that she could make a mess on without reservation. She was, like a caterpillar, without any restriction that she was conscious of.

Over the following months, Kitty recovered. (Social services do their best to help young mothers like Mary to recover relationship, love and resume responsibility for their child, but it was not successful on this occasion.) I last heard of Kitty when she was ten, healthy, with a well-adjusted loving family.

Children can also need to go back to the earlier stage of freedom from any responsibility when life has gone astray.

John, aged twelve and from an upper middle-class family, was referred for stealing any money he came across. Matters came to a head when it was found that he had stolen money from a local newsagent. There were no apparent untoward events in his life. My advice was that he should not have access to any money that had not been given to him; it was not his responsibility to stop stealing and if any money was stolen the person at fault was the one who had left money about and accessible to John.

I had an irate call from his father that night. He would accept my advice but considered me completely wrong and that John, like all children, should learn to be responsible and trustworthy.

Three weeks later, he phoned to apologize. John was happier and more relaxed than he had been for years. In short, John was no longer responsible for self-containing himself, controlling his 'expansiveness'. Within a few months John became much more responsible and could be trusted again.

In the developmental stage that follows birth (Piaget's sensorimotor), the baby exercises sensation and mobility. Synchronicity with the sounds of its carers at about six months helps it to start acquiring speech and by two years there may be bowel and bladder control; however, there can be wide differences. Continence aside, the infant is apertic in the first two years, without any responsibility to self-contain but enjoying the warmth and praise when it responds to, copies, others. It has no responsibility for its own care or safety.

Around the age of two years a toddler begins a change from egocentricity to self-containing. (In this third stage in insect life, a pupa is in a self-contained or separated condition from the environment whilst the dramatic physiological processes to become an imago – butterfly/moth – take place.) In primates this period is used to shape the generally recedic condition to absorb the ways that adults behave in order (like young chimpanzees) to gain acceptance and success in the community in which they will live. Over a fairly prolonged period, children learn to recognize emotional 'reflexes' in others and the response of third parties to those involuntary displays.

Infants and adolescents are most concerned with themselves; adolescents in particular are determined to decide for themselves which platform/mode they are going to operate from. Children in the intervening self-containing period are in effect subjugated to their social environment, the parents, family and group that they live with and who determine which apertic or recedic platform the environment is to be assessed and acted upon.

CHAPTER 14

TRANSITION

Disorder is more likely in any system during a metamorphic change, so it is not surprising that it can occur in the transition during the months or years of maturing from an infant to a child.

It is hard for anyone to relinquish an established freedom and to change attitude. No one likes to give up privilege, the freedom to be as we wish, freedom to make our own decisions rather than submitting to the decisions of others.

We are all 'shocked' if we have to change our perceptions from our personal beliefs; for example, if we discover a much-admired acquaintance is addicted to drugs or that a friend we always thought had the same views as oneself (Brexit Leaver or Remainer) has opposite convictions.

If the experience is a shock to us, it is much more intense and potentially destabilizing for an infant not yet ready to accept a perception imposed by mother that differs from its own. When synchrony of the hospitable/inhospitable perception – of the nature of change – can no longer be depended upon.

I can recall such an event. Between two and three years old, I was lifted up by my mother to watch my father take my cot apart and replace it with a proper bed. They were pleased with what they had bought and that it was another step forward in their child's life.

'There,' my mother said. 'Isn't that great, a grown-up bed for you. You don't have to sleep in the cot any more.' In short, a perception was being imposed on me when I didn't feel I wanted change, did not want to lose familiar, protective surroundings.

I believe it remained in my mind because it was the first time I registered a different attitude in my mother to myself. Others have related similar occasions when their perceptions and their mother's attitude first failed to coincide. One recurrent history is that of being introduced, completely unprepared, to a baby brother or sister and being told: 'It's just what you said you wanted!'

The fact that the challenging experience is remembered, when many other memories are not retained, supports a contention that the **first asynchrony between mother and child is a significant experience**.

The difficult transition period has an informal label: the terrible twos.[1]

> '"The terrible twos" is a normal stage in a child's development
> in which a toddler can regularly rebound between reliance
> on adults and a newly burgeoning desire for independence.
> [See comment below] It is a stage that most toddlers will go
> through in varying degrees. At one moment, the child may
> cling to you desperately and, in the next, run away from you
> in a screaming rage. Understanding the terrible twos can help
> you not only cope with these behaviours but find ways to
> better deal with them without anger or aggression.'

Although mood changes and temper tantrums usually begin about the age of two, they can start before the first birthday. The behaviour is not simply defiance but Vincent Iannelli proposes that the toddler is trying to express independence without the communication skills to do so. He notes that responding with anger prolongs the behaviour.

COMMENT: In the context of this work, the struggle to gain independence arises much later. At this stage a 'terrible two toddler'

---

[1] Comment can be found online at 'Very well family', https://www.verywellfamily.com/terrible-twos-and-your-toddler-2634394

is internally driven to avoid surrendering the infantile position, the freedom to determine life for itself. The 'acting out' behaviour may well be frustration at being unable to relax and accept that 'Mother knows best'.

In addition, the complexity of the transition period makes its progression so fragile that it is susceptible to lifelong dysfunctions: autism and a little later ADHD.

> From Wikipedia: **Autism** is a developmental disorder
> characterized by troubles with social interaction and
> communication and by restricted and repetitive behaviour.
> Parents usually notice signs in the first two or three years
> of their child's life. These signs often develop gradually,
> though some children with autism reach their developmental
> milestones at a normal pace and then worsen.[2]

In summary, autism is caused by a combination of genetic and environmental factors. Risk factors include certain infections during pregnancy such as rubella as well as valproic acid, alcohol or cocaine use during pregnancy.

Recent research supports an association of autism with a failure to develop synchronicity or its loss.[3] The research was reported both in the press and on television.

In short, engaging in synchronous communication led to lasting improvement in the child's ability when it had symptoms of autism. I was particularly impressed by one mother who reported on television that she had had most success by allowing her child to lead (i.e. be in the hierarchically superior position).

---

[2] https://en.wikipedia.org/wiki/Autism
[3] 'Parent-mediated social communication therapy for young children with autism: long-term follow-up of a randomized controlled trial', A. Pickles, A. Le Couteur, K. Leadbitter, E. Salomone et al. was published in *The Lancet*, 25 October 2016. The parent therapy to 'enhance dyadic interaction' (parental synchronous response to child communication during interaction) mediated 71% improvement in child communication.

It is possible that separation, not social interaction, is the default position in human and animal life. It avoids any need to change one's established perception of the nature of the social or material environment to fit in, synchronize with others.

> From Wikipedia: **Attention deficit hyperactivity disorder (ADHD)** is a mental disorder of the neurodevelopmental type. It is characterized by problems paying attention, excessive activity, or difficulty controlling behaviour which is not appropriate for a person's age. The symptoms appear before a person is twelve years old, are present for more than six months, and cause problems in at least two settings (such as school, home, or recreational activities).[4]

When children have problems paying attention it may result in poor school performance. Although it causes impairment, particularly in modern society, many children with ADHD have a good attention span for tasks they find interesting. Despite being the most commonly studied and diagnosed mental disorder in children and adolescents, the cause is unknown but most research is directed towards elucidating what is presumed to be a biochemical imbalance.

* * *

In this concept, autism correlates with a failure to establish or retain synchrony. ADHD correlates with a failure to establish or retain acceptance of hierarchical order.

The age when infants are susceptible to autism and slightly later to the onset of ADHD reflect the evolutionary timing of the development of synchrony and of hierarchical acceptance in this concept. It may also be relevant that because ADHD arises after synchrony it is not as rooted in our 'psyche' and as irreversible as autism. Hierarchical positioning is not present in all animals or even

---

[4] https://en.wikipedia.org/wiki/Attention_deficit_hyperactivity_disorder

in all mammals but it is critical for young chimpanzees to accept learning and absorb the reflex responses of others to understand how to navigate their social environment.

The characteristics of autism can be complicated by compensatory phenomena. Just as the hearing of a blind person can become more acute than the sighted, so those with autism may exhibit extraordinary skills. Eleven-year-old Michael knew the year that every model of every make of car was introduced and the dates of every modification.

Children with ADHD have won the battle to retain infant egocentric rejection of hierarchy, but keeping the adult 'out of the driving seat', i.e. being responsible for their own lives, leaves them insecure. Filling their time with infant sensorimotor activity can keep that insecurity at bay. Although they would be expected to exacerbate the excessive activity, stimulant amphetamine-like drugs are prescribed and ameliorate the condition. There is debate about their contradictory effect. In my opinion, as stimulants heighten sensory awareness they diminish the drive for sensory stimulus. It can be compared to satisfying a wish to see an object more clearly with a magnifying glass.

CHAPTER 15

THE SELF-CONTAINING YEARS

When there is a successful transition from infancy, children very largely relinquish responsibility for interpreting the nature of events and the character of other people; it is a time when class, race and religious prejudices are instilled. He or she submits to most parental decisions and to the example of those 'in loco parentis', which can be confused with every older person, including elder siblings. When an elder sibling smokes, for example, a child is more likely to take up smoking than if their parents smoke.

The other half of the contract is that the actions of parents or those in their place should always be in the child's interest and that the child has confidence in that circumstance. In addition to giving and encouraging affection, a parent has to suffer pain at times[1] or oppose (which may be difficult) a dominant spouse when their behaviour is oppressive upon or belittling their son or daughter.

In many children's lives the relationship with parents goes well. Unhappily, unusual experiences can distort it.

---

[1] I was asked to see Ted, twelve, and Tom, ten, whose behaviour antagonized everyone in the small town in which they lived. Every car and greenhouse was a target for their stone throwing, and they were threatened with being taken into care. When I asked their mother what she did when they were found to have caused damage, she replied that she punished them severely and I asked further what happened then. 'They cry an awful lot.' 'And then?' 'It makes me feel sorry for them so I give them sweets to stop them crying.' Unfortunately, if children are not allowed to be unhappy when they should be, through their behaviour, their behaviour will never change.

Stephen, aged ten, had been a happy, bright, clean and tidy boy but in the eighteen months before coming to see me, he had lost interest in everything, including himself. He was referred because he had stolen from another family.

I learnt that Stephen had suffered from leukaemia at the age of five and was treated successfully through prolonged and very painful treatment. It was emphasized to me how incredibly good he had been in putting up with the pain and that he had been much praised for doing so.

It was unfortunate that because Stephen had been so praised he could not show how 'inhospitable', how wretched he found life at that time. He subsequently rationalized that he was right to suffer pain because he was unworthy, which led to a loss of self-esteem and the belief that he would never succeed at anything and that it was useless trying.

After Stephen and his parents gained insight and understanding, Stephen recovered his former personality in a few weeks.

I know from my experience that it is very easy for boys to feel unworthy. They know their father would like them to show manliness, to succeed at sport, etc. When it is not attained, first there is a feeling of not having tried enough, then hopelessness at ever achieving it, followed by feelings of inadequacy and eventually of not being the child that was wanted.

* * *

In the contract that 'parents are there for the child', children can accept that harsh discipline is imposed to induce them to be socially acceptable, but they can also sense when the disciplinarian is using punishment for his/her own satisfaction. They are also aware that sexual abusers are using them for self-satisfaction and the only way such events can be rationalized, as with Stephen, is to believe that one is without value, which predisposes one to lifelong loss of self-esteem.

Leaving it to adults to assess the environment and make decisions upon it, for children in the self-containing stage, does not mean that children have no opportunity to exercise freedom to make their own decisions; however, freedom needs to be monitored by responsible adults.

A child patient of mine was left with other five- and six-year-olds on their own in a garden whilst their mothers enjoyed tea inside the house. Unfortunately, they had their own tea party and fed each other laburnum pods, which are highly poisonous. They just survived after urgent stomach washouts. Children a year or two older often know that some berries can be poisonous. Allowing children the freedom to be on their own and to make their own decisions changes with the age of the child.

Young children cannot choose to be in the self-containing condition, to be receptive to learning, for themselves. The responsibility rests with the adult to create an environment where the child can acquire essential social knowledge and skills. Unfortunately, many diverse influences can interrupt parental or adult motivation to determine and to display what mode is most appropriate and advantageous for their child. Parents cannot, for example, expect children to accept the imposition of a recedic attitude whilst freely indulging themselves.

It should be obvious that children need intermittent relief from being recedic, which should be neither severe nor extended. Regular playtime is necessary but that unfortunately causes its own difficulties when rebound from self-containing provokes excessive assertiveness and harassment of vulnerable companions in the playground.

A not uncommon childhood phenomenon illustrates one of the management problems. Most contented and secure children are appropriately cooperative and self-controlled. From time to time parents may arrange a holiday, a party, a festive occasion and include their children in the happy anticipation and excitement. When the occasion takes place, parents can be dismayed to find that their child's behaviour has changed to selfishness and bad manners.

Unfortunately, in emphasizing enjoyment of the coming event, the parents have advertised that it will be exceptionally 'hospitable'.

The child cannot help unconsciously interpreting that message as an environment to be freely enjoyed without restriction.

There are several parenting traits that do not help children. One is weakness, when a parent wants other people to put hierarchical positioning of the child in place for them. They claim it is the schoolteacher's responsibility to teach a child to behave, for example. There are other abdications of parental responsibility. A parent may not want to be a 'nasty person', whilst others do not want to make the effort. Some want to avoid any responsibility for making decisions. I was asked to see David, aged eleven, because he had become bad-tempered and depressed. I found that he was being pressed to decide which school he should go to when he needed his parents (academics who disagreed with each other) to make the decision. One burdensome but common decision a child can be called upon to make is to choose which parent to live with when they are separating. This can end in the child rejecting both parents.

Child psychiatrists and GPs can be pressed to become the substitute parent. 'You tell him, doctor. You tell him to behave himself; he will do it for you.'

The infant freedom persists in a small number of children; at four and five they can still be in the 'driving seat' in their lives, determined to behave as they wish. Such children need to be shown and know that ultimately the parents can impose their will without deprecating language, condemning or physically punishing. One successful technique is for the parent to use a suitable opportunity when the child is misbehaving, such as pointlessly damaging a piece of furniture, and when there is time and no audience. The child should be told that it will be held on the settee or bed next to the parent so that it can no longer continue to damage. The threat will immediately exacerbate the child's behaviour. The child should be picked up and sitting down with it, held around the waist. It will probably kick, scratch, bite, spit and assault the parent in any way it can think of. Apart from continuing to hold the child the parent should ignore it, not reprimanding or trying to persuade the child to stop but after a minute or two when its energy has started to ebb say: 'I am going to count to ten and then let you down.' Fury always returns as the child is desperate to show itself that it can determine what is going to happen.

After counting, the exhausted child can be released and the parent leave the room so that the child has no stimulation to continue to rebel. The exercise seldom has to be repeated more than once or twice in the next few days, nor should it be. It is painful for parent and child to suffer but in the majority of occasions such children settle and quite quickly become more loving. Children who do not learn to self-contain remain unhappy, often unhealthy and become socially dysfunctional adults.

Ian was referred to me aged ten because he was overweight. He had absolute control of his life including when and what he ate. I learnt that since infancy his diet had consisted solely of cornflakes with milk, a bottle of undiluted Ribena and at least a quarter-pound bar of milk chocolate every day.

Control can be administered extremely inappropriately. One very young infant was ordered by her father to shut the kitchen door for him. She crawled on hands and knees across the room to do as she was told. The father was proud of his achievement in 'training'. I noticed that in her progress across the floor the infant kept out of her father's reach. The child was later taken into care.

But the opposite extreme, absence of supervision, can also be profoundly destructive. The social services once asked me to see Richard, aged eleven, to try to identify the best placement for him. Reports recorded that he had been coerced by near neighbours into enjoying diverse sexual activity and drugs every weekday during his primary school years. Richard had gone into school at the front entrance and straight out at the back. Children's homes could not contain him and no unit would accept him because of his propensity for perverting other children.

Interviewing the mother, I asked, 'Didn't you ever think that something was wrong?'

'I cannot bear thinking that anything is going wrong in my life, so I never do.'

I asked Richard's father if he felt responsible. 'No.'

'Why not?'

'He is responsible for what he does. Everyone is responsible for what they do.'

'Even as a newborn?'

'Er, no.'

'When are they responsible?'

'When they can talk.'

'As soon as children can talk?'

'Yes.'

I would be surprised, but very relieved, to hear that Richard has escaped the consequences of his experiences and avoided imprisonment for rape or paedophilia.

CONSTRUCTIVE EXPERIENCES
AND SOME THAT ARE LOST

Playing board games as a family can provide useful experience. Learning that being recedic in games like Monopoly can be more successful in playing than being continually apertic, and that saving resources can be profitable, is helpful. Discovering that cooperation may help to win is also useful, and opportunities to beat Mum and Dad encourage self-esteem. Unfortunately, some parents find it difficult to give up their hierarchical position in any way and just as a child is going to beat them at chess, squash or another sport they find reasons to avoid playing.

The drive for synchrony with parents means that many children want to copy their activities and their clothes. Before the Industrial Revolution most parents worked at or near home and children could see their skills and the work they undertook. They would also see that others admired craft skills and how self-esteem can be acquired. Those opportunities were lost in the 19th century and largely replaced by finding self-esteem in becoming rich. Even that does not appear to be appealing enough in the 21st century, where multi-millionaires compete to become television celebrities.

For a modern teenager, only two avenues appear to bring success and self-esteem: sport, mainly as a footballer, or becoming an entertainer. Success in either can only be guaranteed for a very few. The chance of an occupation that brings self-esteem appears remote if not impossible to many children. The position can be eased by being an accepted member of a group or made much worse by isolation and degrading comments by peers.

It is easy to turn to hating and punishing oneself and one's body for failing to be successful, failing to be good enough. Cut it, starve it or completely separate from it – in suicide.

CHAPTER 16

MOVING TO ADULTHOOD

The transition through puberty into adulthood, accompanied by physical and behavioural change, is another unstable period. Adolescents move away from acceptance that their parents determine the character of events and best response. The transition cannot happen without some rejection of parental attitudes and interests.

The degree of rejection varies: some teenagers in total rejection leave home and walk away from everything the parent is attached to. Most detach from just some parts of their beliefs. Paradoxically, rejection of the parent can be because they have not pursued their convictions strongly enough. Vegetarian parents may be rejected, for example, either by their children becoming meat eaters or by becoming vegan, more totally committed.

A postgraduate student was referred to me because he refused to complete the work that remained – of less than a day in length – for him to gain his PhD. He commented that once you have a PhD, that's what you are, you cannot get rid of it. To the best of my knowledge he never undertook the work and it was not my place to try to persuade him to do so. Both his parents were senior lecturers.

One insightful mother said to me, 'I wish that like our neighbours we had pushed sport or another interest at our children. My neighbours made their children take part in sports in every available moment. Now in their late twenties, they don't spend a minute on sports but have settled lives and very amiable relationships with their parents.'

During childhood, many children wish to dress like their parents and ceasing to do so is a convenient way of rejecting them – but it does mean if a mother bought her clothes at M&S, her daughter is unlikely to want to do the same. Each generation needs its own music, own interests and own styles to separate from parental perceptions.

Adolescence could be compared, especially for boys, to stopping a programme and beginning again. Reinstituting elemental behaviours: time, sensory awareness in colour and music, synchrony with own age and hierarchical exercising – in the driving seat of his/her life whether he or she wants to be or not, and with many anxieties about competence to be there. Biologically, the redirection is necessary to stop individuals being clones of their parents.

CHAPTER 17

SLEEP AND DREAMING

Before moving to mental disorders, the servicing activity of sleep and dreaming needs to be discussed.

In this work it has been contended that humans, like insects in their egg and pupa stages, experience self-contained recedic periods so that all available resources can be allocated to physiological and psychological growth, relieved of monitoring and responding to the external environment.

The phenomenon is replicated on a smaller scale during the 24-hour diurnal rhythm when self-containment in sleep allows our physiology to 'catch up', metabolizing nutrients and restoring biochemical balances. It helps to ensure that our physiology fulfils all the demands made upon it. One physiological necessity, for example, is to rid ourselves of excess nitrogen by converting it into urea and excreting it. If the process fails we become ill; patients with kidney failure need to be dialysed (in other words, their physiological condition serviced) three times a week.

Our interpretation of and response to events that happen to us during the day are just as complex as our physiology and need similar care to regain 'homeostasis' (page 17) of our behavioural system when nothing else is happening, when we are asleep.

The experiences that we sustain during the day can be compared to a busy police station. Everything is noted, events inside and outside the station, interviews, information coming in and decisions taken. There is a need at the end of the day to make sure that records have been made, cross-referenced, consideration given to whether an event matches a similar one in the past, filed in the right place, quite possibly in several places. Before computers were available the need was best accomplished by an overnight clerk, because it is only possible to carry out when nothing else is happening, nothing is coming in.

Our minds are as complex as a police station and we have a similar need to resolve the significance of every experience and file it.

The process takes place as dreaming and, just as our physiology breaks up compounds to get rid of an excess of nitrogen, one action of dreaming is to depressurize outstanding events and to release any excess of oscillation and resulting arousal. Its success is evident in much greater ease after a night's sleep when the emotional intensity of both joyful and untoward events is diminished.

Dreams can be said to resemble the activities of the overnight clerk, resolving a day's fears and excitement, collating past and present events and influences on the future. Servicing a system to keep it running smoothly.

The vital need to dream is apparent when we are prevented from sleep and dreaming: our memory deteriorates and we become disorientated.

CHAPTER 18

DISORDER

Genetic influences and stressful experiences can cause a suscepti-bility to mental illness but the actual dysfunctions are currently believed to be biochemical imbalances. The presumption has been given impetus through new and sophisticated instruments and tech-niques that allow researchers to track biochemical activity as it takes place. Psychiatrists could be said to be waiting with impatience for a 'breakthrough' to take place.

Possibly the most striking feature of mental illness is that the common disorders reach epidemic proportions in human society, but do not appear to occur naturally in animal or even mammalian life. Animals show anxiety or an urge to separate when pursued, and hibernation is a separation similar to depression, but those rational responses do not continue beyond the events that have aroused them.

An obvious conclusion is that although our primate evolution has brought intelligence and ability, it has also brought functional fragility.

Before considering the common disorders, there are behaviours that can so far overstep what is acceptable in civilized society that they become antisocial and occasionally criminal.

PREJUDICE

In many circumstances, and especially in old age, we find familiar places, foods and decorations the most desirable, in this concept the most hospitable. Whether we choose what is familiar or not, we also fall into a habit of placing what we like in hierarchical order. But there is an opposite pole, another side of the coin.

In our generally hospitable environment, our awareness of what is or could be *in*hospitable has little exercise. It was indicated earlier (page 36) that every trait needs to be exercised and in exercising the trait both 'poles' may occasionally need to be expressed. There is unconscious satisfaction, fulfilling a need, when we find an object, person or race to which we can attach the inhospitable 'classification'. We then know who, where and what 'the inhospitable' is so we can relax for most of the time, when there is no evidence of their presence. Chimpanzees find an inhospitable target in Colobus monkeys that they hunt (as on television) like an excited mob. The species are similar but not quite the same as themselves. The phenomenon is similar to a human rejection of others – the disabled, the mentally ill, other races – who are 'not quite' the same. There is often a more acute rejection of 'not quite the same' than that shown to the completely alien.

This reflects the reality that a circumstance that is slightly asynchronous (e.g. a piece of music, a combination of colour shades) is more discomfiting than the introduction of a completely different tune or colour.

Adding momentum to an allocation of inhospitableness can convert it to what we call hatred. And just as it is invigorating to be in a community united in an apertic mood, such as a music festival, so it is invigorating to hate together. As with the escalating synchrony of music festivals, joining with those who have similar feelings energizes oscillation, inflaming emotion.

MISCHIEF

Chimpanzees and human children are accepted into the community through self-containing to the expectations of the group. This continues into adulthood, where for the most part having a recedic attitude is pervasive and apertism is relatively inhibited. But, again in accord with a drive for both poles of an attribute to be exercised, we can indulge apertism in provoking responses in others that range from irritation to dismay.

In my experience everyone can commit mischief, preferably clandestinely. For example, making derogatory comments about a third party that we know will be passed on, deliberately unsettling other drivers, 'accidentally' breaking something and in many, many other ways. The internet has made it too easy to be mischievous, to be able to deride and bully fellow school pupils.

I misdiagnosed the phenomenon before I comprehended it. The mother of a child who had been referred to me asked for assistance to stop herself shoplifting. She said she couldn't help it. She didn't need what she had stolen but it gave her a thrill (or satisfying oscillation), as mischief does. Groping for a formula, I suggested that she was insufficiently occupied, she needed to take up an alternative interest. That did not happen but her behaviour improved, possibly because her confession and my lack of condemnation removed excitement in the activity.

One malign habit is enjoying mischief by proxy, enjoying the suppressed irritation and discomfort an uncontrolled child's behaviour arouses in others. The hallmark expression is: 'You don't mind, do you, he's only a child.' Some dog owners also enjoy allowing their dog to jump up on anyone. 'It's all right, it's never hurt anyone.' Further mischief by proxy.

There is a phenomenon labelled 'intrusive thoughts' that may be related to mischief.

> From Wikipedia: An **intrusive thought** is an unwelcome involuntary thought, image, or unpleasant idea that may become an obsession, is upsetting or distressing, and can feel difficult to manage or eliminate… Intrusive thoughts, urges, and images are of inappropriate things at inappropriate times, and generally have aggressive, sexual, or blasphemous themes.[1]

---

[1] https://en.wikipedia.org/wiki/Intrusive_thought

Most of us would be reluctant to acknowledge that we had weird 'intrusive thoughts' even to ourselves and much less so to another person; consequently, it is difficult to know how common intrusive thoughts are.

It is possible that intrusive thoughts arise when there has been a need to be restrained, continually recedic, for others and there is no avenue for 'mischief' or rebellion of any kind.

It was no accident that the author Robert Louis Stevenson chose medicine as Jekyll's profession in Dr Jekyll and the archetypal mischief-maker Mr Hyde. If we have to strongly self-contain to one group, such as patients for doctors or passengers for air pilots, the maximum satisfaction arises from destabilizing that particular group. In an extreme example, Dr Shipman murdered his patients and probably gained most reward from the resulting incomprehension of their relatives.

Those who are seen to care for others are usually the last to be suspected of mischief in its many forms.

Immature 'satisfactions' disrupt the lives of individuals and communities.

CHAPTER 19

PERSONALITY DISORDER

Personality disorder is sometimes called borderline disorder because it is on the border between temperamental behaviour and neurosis or illness.

In this concept, personality disorder arises from a failure of behavioural proprioception: from a failure to be aware, to know the temperament or mood that one is in during social events (page 40). It is particularly important in responding to children's behaviour.

Behavioural proprioception, automatic consciousness of one's position in the social group, is present in animal hierarchies from chickens to wolf packs. It needs to be a more adaptable and finely developed resource when triadic thinking in chimpanzee and in human lives complicates naturalization (i.e. fitting in with a constantly shifting community). Having behavioural proprioception and responding to it – like listening to tentative whispers – leads to being accepted and granted the privileges of being part of a community.

The attribute is cultivated through experience in the social group, learning from parents, and particularly the mother's body language, facial expression and tone of vocalizations during her contact with others. It helps if both parents show consistent, united attitudes – and confuses when they do not.

I think my first lesson in hierarchical awareness occurred (aged four) when I recognized the deference that my mother showed to the doctor who visited me when I had mumps.

Identifying 'personality disorder' (PD) as a specific condition is a challenge to academic psychiatrists.

> From Wikipedia: Definitions include every psychiatric symptom but lacking the severity that would place those affected in the more recognized and serious disorders. Essentially, those affected show unstable personal emotions and chaotic behaviour towards others through excessive sensitivity to events and distorted perceptions of social interactions.[1]

Its prevalence in the general community was largely unknown until surveys starting from the 1990s were published:

> In 2008 the median rate of diagnosable PD was estimated at 10.6 per cent based on six major studies across three nations. In other words, when one in ten are associated with high use of services, it is a major public health concern that calls for more attention by researchers and clinicians.

The cause of personality disorder is sought and debated in many studies, all of which disclose a close association between damaging experiences in childhood and developing the condition:

> From Wikipedia:

> (i) A study of 600 male college students, averaging 30 years of age, elicited both a history of abuse in those with the disorder and that the severity of abuse was associated with more intractable symptoms.

> (ii) In another study, efforts were taken to match

---

[1] https://en.wikipedia.org/wiki/Personality_disorder

retrospective reports of abuse with a clinical population
that had demonstrated psychopathology from childhood to
adulthood. It was later found that they had experienced abuse
and neglect.

But sexual and physical abuse and neglect were not the only predis-
posing experiences:

> (iii) Researchers asked 793 mothers and children if they or
> their mothers had screamed at them as children and told
> them that they did not love them or threatened to send them
> away. Children who had experienced such verbal abuse were
> three times as likely as other children to have borderline,
> narcissistic, obsessive-compulsive or paranoid personality
> disorders in adulthood.
>
> The sexually abused group demonstrated the most
> severe symptoms. Officially verified physical abuse showed
> an extremely strong correlation with the development of
> antisocial and impulsive behaviour. However, pathological
> behaviour following childhood neglect showed some
> improvement in adulthood.

Children of parents with personality disorders are more likely to
suffer from the same condition but whether that follows a genetic
predisposition or the consequences of erratic parenting is uncertain.

The condition, as noted above, improves with age – which can
bring psychological maturity.

CHAPTER 20

PSYCHOPATHY AND PTSD

Two completely different phenomena that derive from archaic responses:

> From Dictionary.com: **Psychopathy**
> A mental disorder in which an individual manifests amoral and antisocial behaviour, lack of ability to love or establish meaningful personal relationships, extreme egocentricity, failure to learn from experience, etc.[1]

Children who suffer acute deprivation, hunger, isolation, frequently accompanied by physical abuse in the first weeks after birth, are susceptible to lasting psychopathic traits for the rest of their lives. The most affected children have been labelled 'feral'.

The deprivation undermines any ability to move from the biological level of 'competitive survival' to seek self-esteem and self-respect. Those affected have no respect for themselves, have no respect for anyone else, have no wish to join in synchrony, or in friendship at any depth. Other people become opportunities for exploitation.

In recent years, those who have shown a ruthless determination to dominate in business, politics and the professions have been called psychopathic.

---

[1] https://www.dictionary.com/browse/psychopathy

Psychopathy is either an involuntary retention of acting at the level of survival of the fittest – or a voluntary choice.

From Wikipedia: **Post-traumatic stress disorder**
PTSD is a mental disorder that can develop after a person is exposed to a traumatic event such as sexual assault, warfare, traffic collisions, or other threats on a person's life.
Symptoms may include disturbing thoughts, feelings, or dreams related to the events and last for more than a month after the event.[2]

In the initial interpretation of 'response to change' in this concept (page 16), it was asserted that the immediate response to an event was related to the volume or quantity of the environmental change. Overwhelming events trigger an immediate compulsion to completely separate from the situation. If an individual is unable to separate or find a way out, they become physically and mentally paralysed, unable to move on. The physical self may start to move again, but the sentient self, like a needle stuck on a record, has not been able to separate and relives the experience again and again.

It is difficult to know how those suffering PTSD from a devastating event can be helped to recover. Reliving the event in psychotherapy has not always helped. It may be that therapists have encouraged focus upon the recall of details rather than facilitating a cathartic – tearful – separation emotion.

In the small number of cases that I have seen, it was important for the individual to have an opportunity to recount every detail of the event on one occasion, to a professional, outside of friends and family and to have their perception of what happened accepted as the reality, with acceptance evident in the emotional reflexes of the therapist but without verbal comment. The person affected needs to feel that the listener is in synchrony with the emotions that they sustained. Any

---

[2] https://en.wikipedia.org/wiki/Posttraumatic_stress_disorder

interjection, even saying 'that was terrible', means that the listener is 'painting' their own picture of the event, not living the actuality. Subsequently, those that I have seen recover do so by replacing the disordering events with as normal and filled a life as possible.

ANXIETY

Whenever there is an event, we experience arousal similar to the cellular oscillation that is stimulated by every change in the external environment. We respond to it and our arousal is abated.

The experience can be compared to meeting a dog that barks: either a welcoming barking that is open to our approach, inviting a friendly tickle, or aggressive barking, intruding upon our freedom to walk where we wish, causing us to withdraw to an alternative path.

In having gained intelligence, we can anticipate such an event, summon up images that create the arousal we would feel at the actual event. Unfortunately, in that anticipation we extend events and feel more intense arousal than may actually occur. We readily envisage, for example, being badly bitten by the dog.

We call that arousal anxiety, which can become amplified into an overwhelming, even a chronic condition.

Professor Ian Robertson's experiment (page 14) suggests that anxious arousal is only given character, of threat or of thrilling excitement, by how we choose to interpret the event. In the context of this work, we should approach change in an apertic, rather than a recedic mode. It does not account for inherent prejudice to height, deep water and to fire, for example. We do not have a choice when they present themselves. They induce an instant animal-like arousal: fear.

Anxiety is more intrusive in recedic periods such as depression and old age, whilst the apertic young are less concerned about what might or might not happen to them. It should be recognized that some control their thoughts like Richard's mother (page 80): 'I cannot bear thinking that anything is going wrong in my life, so I never do.'

Anxiety is a natural emotion and not of itself a dysfunction. It cannot be surprising that as we are intelligent and can determine so much more of our lives than other animals, we run through and repetitively imagine anticipated events. When anxiety is exacerbated, either through the seriousness of an event or through repetitive experiences, it acquires momentum, is difficult to displace and can make us less competent.

DECISION-MAKING

Our awareness of time and the ability to foresee future possibilities brings with it the ability to choose the best response to a prospective event, in short to make decisions.

However, in order to have that opportunity we have to move away from the animal survival habit. We have to suppress the inherent urge to act immediately when change occurs. The continued suppression of what is for animals a life-preserving reflex leads to a condition we call 'stressed', made worse by our ability to accept a 'queue' of decisions. The latter facility is evident in Professor Sophie Scott's (page 5) observation that, unlike animals, we can accept and store a series of instructions, each of which involves a decision.

Whenever change occurs, whenever there is an event, the hindbrain is the first site to show arousal. Impulses are transmitted backwards and forwards to other parts of the brain before a decision and response are resolved.

Human decisions are much more complex than those of the great apes. But apart from the forebrain, our cerebral resource and functions are not significantly different to great ape brains. It would not be surprising if the gateway, whether it is in the hindbrain or elsewhere, could be overtaxed.[3]

---

[3] The genetic difference between humans and chimps is less than 2% (Wikipedia, https://en.wikipedia.org/wiki/Human_evolutionary_genetics).

When we have made a decision, when we no longer have to carry it 'at the back of our mind', the relief feels as if 'a weight has been taken off our shoulders' (or our heads).

Personal decisions are as demanding to the individual as the critical decisions that a cardiac surgeon or prime minister has to resolve. Single mothers are particularly burdened in having to act on their own.

Some learn to limit choice in order to diminish the burden of decisions. It is said that President Obama reduced his choice of suits to two and had the same evening snack every day.

It was noted on page 35 that a 'lower' hierarchical position diminishes the necessity to make decisions. It occurs in lobsters and crayfish when the group allows one individual to lead and decide which way to go. Many soldiers refuse promotion and in civilian life many reject offers to become managers. We avoid the stress of responsibility for making decisions that affect other people's lives.

Although we may decline management responsibilities or avoid making decisions for other people, it does not mean that we readily accept someone else's decisions on the hospitable/inhospitable nature of an event.

We strive to have our own perception and to arrive at our own decision. The independent trait is particularly evident when language is used to convey a personal[4] opinion: if I give an item of news or information (i.e. knowledge about the environment or part of it) to another person and then hear them repeat it to a third party, it is *never* precisely retold. Slightly different expressions are used that give the item a different 'spin'. If I challenge the reteller, they reply that they are just choosing words that they are used to. In reality, the reteller is inserting their independent perception, most often raising or lowering the advantage/disadvantage quality of the event. The phenomenon is recorded by Anthony Powell in *Temporary Kings*:

---

[4] In the past two decades, others have 'shared' information with me. It is a euphemism that pretends the informer is doing me a favour and attempts to diminish my rejection when they are often satisfying their own needs.

'An extension of that fact is that every story that one hears has to be adjusted, in the mind of the listener to the prejudices of the teller, in practice most listeners increasing, reducing, discarding much of what they have been told.'[5] Powell, conceitedly, does not recognize that he, the listener and subsequently the reteller, is the one who is inserting his own prejudice.

The human compulsion to make independent decisions is reluctantly suppressed when we accept advice or the decisions of others.

It is evident that although human intelligence has brought immense advantage it has also brought the disadvantages of damaging anxiety and being stressed. Both carry the risk of more serious mental disorder and physical illnesses such as raised blood pressure.

---

[5] Powell, Anthony, *Temporary Kings* (Heinemann Ltd, 1973).

CHAPTER 21

PSYCHIATRIC ILLNESS

In this work I have tried to make sense of behavioural phenomena and dysfunctions connecting together known facts and my own experience. Continuing with that basis it is possible to associate mental illnesses with some of the characteristics of physical illnesses. They relate to diagnosis, to dysfunction and to the consequences of malfunction.

Many physical illnesses have complications and side effects that can confuse the diagnosis. Raised blood pressure, for example, can be caused by renal dysfunction and, as it may be discovered before the renal dysfunction has been identified, it can be mistakenly thought to be the primary disorder. Similarly, it is possible that the incomprehensible behaviour observed in psychosis arises from secondary consequences.

Secondly, whenever a 'working part' is adapted, reorganized to undertake an additional or changed function, it becomes more susceptible to disruption.

The shoulder joint is a typical example. In most quadrupeds the forelimb is used in running and is only required to flex and extend. In the evolution of our species it has become able to flex, extend, abduct away from the body, adduct towards it and to circumrotate. Our wrist joints are similarly adapted; the wrist and shoulder joints suffer dislocation more easily and more frequently than our other joints.

Further, when disruption occurs in any 'working part', there are two common consequences: the function can become erratic, like an unstable shoulder joint, or perform less freely, as with the stiffening of arthritis.

Professor Brian Cox underlined (page 18) that we are constructed from parts that are already available. Our organs and functions have evolved through countless adaptations. One very useful reorganization that biologists admire is adaptation of the first digit to become a prehensile thumb, enabling primates to hold small objects, including tools, very successfully.

The contention is that our cerebral functions are susceptible to disorder because they have been achieved through radical reorganizations. And that even the most dramatic symptoms may be the consequence of secondary disorder. Further, that disorder may result in erratic or retarded function or a mixture of both.[1]

* * *

Psychiatrists have struggled for decades to separate dysfunctions and mental illnesses into specific disorders defined by particular groups of symptoms. There are two official bodies that attempt to fulfil that need.

From The International Classification of Diseases (ICD-10) produced by the World Health Organization (WHO) [*i.e. ten attempts to classify psychiatric conditions – changing every time*]

The Diagnostic and Statistical Manual of Mental Disorders (DSM-5), produced by the American Psychiatric Association (APA) [*i.e. five attempts*]

---

[1] Critics may argue that our brains have evolved through extensive enlargement. That is true. We may have Rolls Royce brains, but they still have to function with the basic structures, the same internal combustion engine as in a Model T Ford.

Both list categories of disorders thought to be distinct types. There have been significant differences in the past but in recent revisions there has been a deliberate attempt to converge the codes. Convergence does not hide the reality that resolving mental illnesses into separate defined conditions has been and continues to be a matter of debate. Nor does it consider that the symptoms used to differentiate the disorders may be the consequences of secondary dysfunction, as suggested above.

Possibly the only consensus that all are agreed upon is that individual resistance to mental illness and the ability to withstand the vicissitudes of life is shaped by the experiences we sustain in childhood and later life and, to a lesser extent, genetic factors.

CHAPTER 22

DEPRESSION

In the earliest stages of life, in this concept, primitive organisms in an apertic state engaged in active exchange with the external environment; the apertic state alternated with the separated recedic condition, which facilitated internal repair and restoration. The efficient alternation combined with biological rhythms to create a stable, diurnal rotation that coincided with the natural environment and continued as an integrated system to our own species.

As hominids evolved to *Homo sapiens* they learnt to preserve and control fire, providing them with light and heat when they wanted it. When cities arose, artificial environments were created. Individuals were no longer tied to the natural timetable and those that adapted and succeeded in the more flexible pattern would have advantage, perpetuating an adaptive trait. When we have flown halfway round the planet, the trait allows us to reset our physiology in one or two days. It is a flexibility that could only be achieved by loosening the long-established unity between the apertic/recedic alternation and biological rhythms.

The change has brought susceptibility to disorder that mirrors common consequences. The balanced rotation of the recedic and apertic states is either retarded, sticking in one phase or the other, causing the conditions we label resistant depression or mania. Or it becomes an unstable bipolar rotation between the two states.

Circumstances can occur that make added demands on the system and cause it to be more susceptible to disruption. They include loss of physiological equilibrium through illness, loss of psychological equilibrium in unemployment, divorce, death of a partner and other inhospitable or untoward events. Although we cannot take ourselves out of depression by arranging hospitable events, some individuals are conscious that an episode threatens and pursue self-assertive displacement behaviour in an attempt to avoid it, which leads to overeating, drinking alcohol, sexual assault or mischief.[1]

In contrast to those indulgent behaviours, a voluntary or involuntary disastrous event may reverse the depressed condition. Many depressed people attempt and commit suicide. Ruth, an intelligent but profoundly affected patient, jumped from a multi-storey car park shortly before I became responsible for her care. She survived the attempt, sustaining many painful fractures, but instantly lost the symptoms of depression. It is possible that reaching the most profound 'separated' state restarts a balanced alternation.

In a very recent publication, *The Inflamed Mind*,[2] Edward Bullmore makes ground-breaking observations. He identifies an association between cytokines that are secreted in inflammation caused by physical infection or injury – and depression. 'The blood concentrations of C-reactive protein and some cytokines are increased in patients with depression' (page 116 of the cited work). In other words, cytokines are raised in some patients with depression whether inflammation is present or not. The discovery raises the possibility that cytokines contribute to depression and that neutralizing them or blocking their production could alleviate the disorder.

However, whatever has caused the inflammation, either injury or infection are 'inhospitable events' and the presence of cytokines in depression may follow its onset rather than cause the condition. The phenomenon appears to me to be a physical response to both physical and psychological inhospitable events, a response that echoes the phenomenon of crying tears, which can happen through

---

[1] Andreas Lubitz, a pilot who is believed to have deliberately crashed a plane full of travellers, showed evidence of depressive episodes.
[2] Bullmore, Edward, *The Inflamed Mind* (Short Books Ltd, 2018).

separating from inhospitable dust in an eye or an overwhelming emotional event (page 63).

* * *

Lithium compounds, regularly used in bipolar disorder, are labelled 'mood stabilizing' drugs. The way in which they work is not understood. However, we might rationally conjecture that in the context of this concept, and like the effect of digitalis compounds upon irregular heart contractions, lithium could stabilize the cyclical rhythm rather than correcting the consequences of its disruption, the changed mood.

When medication fails to alleviate depression, ECT may be used to 'stop the clock', interrupting the malfunction with the hope that a balanced rhythm will emerge.

CHAPTER 23

SCHIZOPHRENIA

The dysfunction that occurs in schizophrenia has not been resolved – quite simply, nobody knows what goes wrong or why. There have been many attempts to make sense of the condition by classifying and defining groups of symptoms in the hope that, like rearranging the pieces of a jigsaw, a rational picture will fall into place.

Two celebrated authors moved away from categorizing mental illness: in *The Myth of Mental Illness* Thomas Szasz argued against labelling people who are 'disabled by living' as mentally ill, and I have listened to R. D. Laing rejecting the 'medical model of mental illness' (Sheffield mid 1980s). Both attracted support but as they offered no coherent alternative, interest has fallen away.

The most frustrating aspect is that, unlike physical illnesses and excepting enlargement of the cerebral ventricles or spaces in schizophrenia, no other physical or consistent biochemical changes have been established in individuals suffering from the condition.

Diagnosis is compiled from the thought and behaviour disorders that are considered to be characteristic of the condition.

From NHS Choices – Changes in thinking and behaviour are the most obvious signs of schizophrenia, but people can experience symptoms in different ways.[1]

---

[1] https://www.nhs.uk/conditions/schizophrenia/symptoms/

The symptoms of schizophrenia are usually classified into one of two categories – positive or negative. Positive symptoms – represent a change in behaviour or thoughts, such as hallucinations or delusions. Negative symptoms – represent a withdrawal or lack of function that you would not expect to see in a healthy person; for example, people with schizophrenia often appear emotionless, flat and apathetic. The condition may develop slowly. The first signs of schizophrenia, such as becoming socially withdrawn and unresponsive or experiencing changes in sleeping patterns, can be hard to identify. This is because the first symptoms often develop during adolescence and changes can be mistaken for an adolescent 'phase'.

Summarized from Wikipedia:

People often have episodes of schizophrenia, during which their symptoms are particularly severe, acute schizophrenia, followed by periods where they experience few or no positive symptoms. Individuals with schizophrenia may experience hallucinations (most reported are hearing voices), delusions (often bizarre or persecutory in nature), and disorganized thinking and speech. The last may range from loss of train of thought, to sentences only loosely connected in meaning, to speech that is incomprehensible and is known as word salad in severe cases. Social withdrawal, sloppiness of dress and hygiene, and loss of motivation and judgment are all common in schizophrenia. There is often an observable pattern of emotional difficulty, for example lack of responsiveness. Impairment in social cognition [in this concept, impaired behavioural proprioception] is associated with schizophrenia, as are symptoms of paranoia. Social isolation commonly occurs. Difficulties in working and long-term memory, attention, executive functioning, and speed of processing also commonly occur. In one uncommon subtype, the person may be largely mute, remain motionless in bizarre postures, or exhibit purposeless agitation, all signs of catatonia. About 30 to 50 per cent of people with schizophrenia fail [or refuse?] to accept that they have an illness or their recommended treatment. Treatment may have some effect on insight. People with schizophrenia often find facial emotion perception to be difficult.[2]

The extract from 'NHS Choices' underlines our preoccupation with classification, differentiating the predominance of hallucinations or apathy into 'positive' and 'negative' forms of psychosis. The Wikipedia author notes that 'individuals *may* experience hallucinations' but marks episodic change.

A different picture unfolds if patients are encouraged to relate the actual experiences they sustain. James Chapman recorded his patients' descriptions of living with schizophrenia:[3]

'Things go too quick for my mind. Everything is too fast and too big for me – too quick to study. Things get blurred and it's like being blind. I can't make them out clearly. It's as if you were seeing one picture one minute and another picture the next. I just stop and watch my feet. If I move everything alters every minute and I have no control over my legs… The sun seemed too big for me and it was coming closer. Everything else seemed to be coming closer and bigger all the time.'

'Everything I see is split up. It's like a photograph that is torn in bits and put together again. If somebody moves or speaks, everything I see disappears quickly and I have to put it together again.'

---

[2] https://en.wikipedia.org/wiki/Schizophrenia
[3] *The British Journal of Psychiatry*, 1966, Vol 112, pp 225–251.

'I have to put things together in my head. If I look at my watch I see the watch, watchstrap, face, hands and so on, then I have got to put that together to get into one piece.'

'I have to build up a picture of someone. If something interrupts me, the picture is not finished. You did it just now. You spoke while I was building up the picture. I was trying to hold on to it and listen to you at the same time. I lost it. You spoke and it faded away.'

'If I do something like going for a drink of water, I've to go over each detail – find cup, walk over, turn tap off, drink it. I keep on building up a picture.'

'There is no depth, but if I take time to look at things I can pick out the pieces like a jigsaw puzzle. Moving is like a motion picture. If you move the picture in front of you changes. The rate of change in the picture depends on speed of walking. If you run you receive the signals at a faster rate. The picture I see is literally made up of hundreds of pieces until I see into the things, I don't know what distance they are away.'

'I go into a daze because I can't concentrate long enough to keep up the conversation.'

'I lose control in conversation then I sweat and shake all over. If somebody is speaking I just let them continue until they are finished – I can't comprehend what they are saying. It's trying to think what they are talking about when they are speaking because I am concentrating so much and trying to listen to what they are saying and I lose track of the conversation.'

The clinician interjected 'Can you hear them?'

'I can hear what they are saying all right. It's remembering
what they have said in the next second that's difficult. It just
goes out of my mind.'

* * *

It may be of value to try to reproduce the experience of those affected
by schizophrenia to help to understand how demanding it can be.

Unlike city living, when I meet someone walking down an
otherwise deserted country lane, greetings are usually exchanged,
often a comment about the weather. If they say 'It's a fine day' to
me, I may reply 'It's been a lovely autumn', concurring with their
perception of a benign environment.

If I were to pass someone who is in an active schizophrenic
episode, they might well appear to be 'emotionless, flat and apathetic'
as described above (page 107) and seemingly half-asleep.

But it should be remembered – if we listen to what they say, rather
than impose our own definitions – they are most likely mentally very
active, trying to resolve their chaotic experiences into manageable order.

Because they are constantly trying to make sense of their lives,
those affected are unable to have a balanced exchange about the
weather. Comments are not neutrally received; if I say, when passing
and intending to be friendly, 'It's a fine day' and it actually penetrates
the schizophrenic preoccupation with resolving their existence, the
statement has to be examined: 'Is it a fine day?' 'Is he telling me how
I should be feeling about the day?' 'Is he testing me to see if I get it
right?' It is not surprising that an affected individual is outwardly
unresponsive.

In trying to make conversation I have added to the sufferer's
confusion and there is a predisposition to believe that when others
have distressed us, as with mischief, it has been intentional.

The 'abnormal' exchange illustrates why patients with schizophrenia are often more settled in lodgings than living with their own
families. The reality is that parents and relatives cannot help but be
dismayed by the erratic social responses and try to encourage, to

nudge, the patient back to reality or normality. In effect, constantly applying value to the patient's behaviour and unavoidably diminishing the patient's self-esteem and confidence in themselves. Some landlords and landladies show exceptional tolerance of the unusual behaviours that sufferers can exhibit.

* * *

The fleeting experiences that James Chapman's patients described could be mistaken for a report of recently experienced dreams.

Earlier in this work it was posited that dreams restore psychological balance as sleep restores the physiological balance. It is possible that severe cerebral disorder activates restorative dreaming even during waking periods to try to regain stability. In such a circumstance, classification of the chaotic thought disorders will not take understanding of the condition any further. In that circumstance the only reliable way forward is to focus on the common characteristics of the condition.

Schizophrenia:

1. appears to be confined to humans;
2. is often associated with higher intelligence;
3. has a moderate inherited predisposition;
4. is often associated with displacing experiences such as losing employment, moving to a foreign environment and the confusion of living in a big city;
5. although the condition often first occurs in the transition state of late adolescence, *schizophrenia is extremely rare, if it ever occurs, in children*;
6. is frequently heralded by disordered sleep.

* * *

Point 1. suggests that schizophrenia arose in our transition from other primates and point 2. could indicate that the reorganization that facilitated our unique human intelligence is flawed.

It is worth returning to that reorganization. To recapitulate (page 44), two trains go to the same destination from different platforms. A slow, cheaper (recedic) train goes from one platform, an expensive (apertic) express from the other. Choice in that situation is limited, polarized and relatively uninformed. On another date the trains are on either side of one platform as if the platforms had been merged. There is much more information (the source of intelligence) available: one train may be more crowded, have food available, hold a friend we want or do not want to meet and many other possibilities. But the more information, the more difficult the choice. There will be rapid fluctuation in choosing between starting one's journey from the apertic side of the platform or the recedic.

Decisions, choosing which platform to use to make one's response from, are demanding enough when the environment is stable and familiar but when we have lost employment or are in a foreign country or the confusion of a large city[4] we are in unfamiliar environments, uncertain about the terminus and even the destination – a situation that arouses frantic fluctuation across the joined-up platforms. A fluctuation that is also loaded with the need to avoid losing self-esteem.

The ease of fluctuation between the two platforms facilitates intelligence and instability – and at the same time it would, like other behavioural characteristics, genetically vary from one individual to another. (We can see similar differences in emotional lability in those around us. Some are volatile whilst others can be described as generally stoical. Characteristics that their children may inherit.)

---

[4] If I, white-haired, travel on the London Underground in the rush hour and have to stand, a Japanese lady might offer me her seat. When I accept it with gratitude, she has been in the right recedic attitude. If I do not wish to see myself as decrepit and refuse the seat it would have been better for her to have remained sitting, unembarrassed by refusal, in the same apertic attitude as the rest of the travellers. Getting attitude correct reassures the individual of their competence in being able to manage the foreign environment; getting it wrong will undermine confidence in the next decision. Uncertainty and indecision make us susceptible to rapid rotation between platforms and increase the difficulty of resolving every new decision.

The most fascinating aspect for me is that although children are subject to anxiety, stress and depression, they are not susceptible to schizophrenia. In this concept they are protected because they do not have responsibility to choose which platform to act from until they reach adolescence (page 70).

Unfortunately, circumstances can diminish that security during the vulnerable period. Researchers from the IOE's Centre for Longitudinal Studies analysed data on more than 6,000 children born in the UK at the turn of the century, who are being followed by the Millennium Cohort Study.

The researchers examined reports of children's mental health at ages three, five, seven, eleven and fourteen, including emotional problems, such as feelings of low mood and anxiety, and behavioural problems, such as acting out and disobedience. They compared information on children who experienced a family split with those who didn't.

A fifth of children in the study saw their parents separate between the ages of three and fourteen. Children whose parents broke up in late childhood and early adolescence, between the ages of seven and fourteen, had, on average, a 16 per cent increase in emotional problems and an 8 per cent rise in conduct issues in the short term. Children whose parents separated earlier, between ages three and seven, were no more likely to experience mental health problems either in the short term or later on, by age fourteen, than those living with both parents.[5] In short, children are more vulnerable during the years that they delegate interpretation of the environment to their parents, than during infancy or adolescence.

Another analogy is appropriate at this point. When I am a passenger in a car I relax completely, confident that the driver is a responsible person who will bring me safely to our destination. If

---

[5] Available online at the UCL Institute of Education homepage and accessed on 6 February 2019 after I was made aware of the publicity for the UCL research in *The Week*, 2 February 2019, under the heading 'Under sevens' divorce resilience' – the journalist missing the significant aspect which the authors recognize, that it is the over sevens' vulnerability that is important.

the driver becomes distracted by an argument with another passenger, I lose my sense of security. If they appear to be about to jump out of the car, I would panic. That is what can happen to children who experience 'a family split'.

* * *

My proposition is that schizophrenia has arisen from a rapid, unstable rotation between apertic and recedic platforms from which every interpretation of change and response is initiated. The instability arises from the reduction of polarization necessary to facilitate the evolution of human intelligence.

Schizophrenia is treated with 'major' tranquillizers; the first modern psychotropic medication was chlorpromazine. Chlorpromazine (from personal experience) removes every motivation, there are *no* decisions to make. There is no interest in maintaining self-esteem. The vegetative condition is unpleasant and it is not surprising that patients are reluctant to accept medication. The dampening reduces activity and usually allows recovery. It is significant (but rational with respect to the damage that can be caused) that the earlier a schizophrenic episode is treated, the better the prognosis.

Anxiety, depression, bipolar and manic disorder show little significant effect upon brain tissue but the cerebral ventricles (open spaces) enlarge in schizophrenia, which means that there must have been loss of physical substance. In other words, schizophrenia is the more mentally and physically damaging condition.

* * *

A logical evolution of behaviour has been set out and it has been proposed that our mental disorders arise from evolutionary functional changes: 1. The period of metamorphic-like infant change **in autism and ADHD**. 2. Movement to excessive adaptability away from the long and close association between apertic (daytime behaviour), recedic (night-time behaviour) and biological rhythms **in depression and manic states**. 3. The subconscious, friable merging of apertic and recedic positions, intrinsic to hominid intelligence, but previously polarized when they had successfully promoted survival throughout evolution, **in schizophrenia.** I labelled appetite enhancement a 'wild card', a joker in the pack. The pursuit of self-esteem is another powerful 'wild card'. Both add oscillatory response to events, often contributing to mental and behavioural instability.

I have made no suggestions as to how mental disorders might be alleviated, though I hope that this concept will help to understand them. We would all like effortless magic (a tablet) to correct disorder but it seems unlikely that a chemical compound will ever succeed more than in relieving symptoms.

Robert Bugler

INDEX

response to change in external
ix, 16, 17, 19, 20, 21, 23, 24,
25, 25n; climatic 17, 31, 44,
45, 46, 50; depression and
103, 104, 105; 'hospitable' or
'inhospitable' 23, 24, 25–6, 28,
29, 32, 36, 43–4, 51, 61, 63, 64,
65, 67, 68, 71, 77, 88, 98, 104,
105; intelligence and 43–4, 46;
primate evolution and 46, 50;
PTSD and 95; schizophrenia
and 110, 111, 112, 112n, 113;
volume of change 23, 23n, 43,
95
every organ and function must be
exercised to continue to exist: 'as
with any biological function, a
lack of use leads to atrophy' 18
evolution 5, 6n, 16, 17, 21, 26;
appetite and 38–9; ADHD/
autism and 74–5, 114; apertic
and recedic behaviour and
28, 29; autonomic nervous
system and 9, 26, 36; cellular
physiology, evolution of response
founded in 24; Darwinian 9,
10, 15; disruption and 100–1;
frontal lobe enlargement and
strive for self-esteem 57–60,
74–5; functional fragility and
74–5, 87, 114–15; intelligence
and 44, 45–54, 87, 114; motility
and 25; natural selection 10–11,
15, 38; primate 44, 45–54,
87; schizophrenia and 115;
sporulation and 28; synchrony
and 31–2, 74
extrovert 30
eye contact 62–3

facial colour 47–8
facial expression 47, 91

fear 14, 63, 86, 96
flagella 17–18, 25
food, sex and appetite 38–9
Freud, Sigmund 14–15
frontal lobe 55–7

Gage, Phineas P. 55–6, 56n
Goodwin, Brian 19–20, 19n

halobacteria 18
Harper, Robert 12, 12n
Harvard Medical School 17
hierarchical positioning 32–5, 33n,
36, 47n, 51, 57, 59, 73, 74–5,
79, 81, 84, 88, 91–2, 98
Hitler, Adolf 34
Hoch, James 27–8, 28n
homeostasis 16, 17, 20, 25, 61, 85
hominids 11, 45, 49–50, 57, 103,
115
Humphrey, N. K. 50n, 52, 52n,
53–4, 54n

Ian (aged ten) 80
Iannelli, Vincent 72–3
instant mode rotation 52–3
insulin secretion 22
intelligence 11, 25n, 35n, 42,
43–4, 45, 46, 50, 50n, 58, 61,
67, 87, 96, 97, 99, 104, 111,
112, 114, 115; primate 49–54,
50n, 51n, 52n, 53n, 54n; social
or emotional 46–9
International Classification of
Diseases (ICD–10) 101
introvert 30
intrusive thoughts 89–90

John (aged twelve) 69–70

Kitty (aged seven months) 68–9
Kleine-Levin Syndrome 36, 36n

Lightning Source UK Ltd.
Milton Keynes UK
UKHW041253271121
394692UK00002B/327